Bonnie Mounayer became interested in the prevention and treatment of back pain after suffering from it herself. In 1984, she helped to set up the Back Shop. She now travels widely to find the best products for the shop, and has established contacts with medical practitioners and manufacturers worldwide. This is her first book.

Susie Wynn-Williams is a chartered physiotherapist and consultant to the Back Shop. She spent eight years working for the National Health Service and in industry, then, after two years working in public relations and advertising, she set up in private practice in London which incorporated work for the Royal Ballet.

Susie Wynn-Williams has served on the Council of the Chartered Society of Physiotherapists and is a member of the National Back Pain Association. This is her second book.

THE BACK SHOP BOOK

BONNIE MOUNAYER
and
SUSIE WYNN-WILLIAMS

Illustrated by SHAUN WILLIAMS

An OPTIMA book

© The Backshop Clinic Ltd 1989

First published in 1989 by
Macdonald Optima, a division of
Macdonald & Co. (Publishers) Ltd

A Member of Maxwell Pergamon Publishing Corporation plc

British Library Cataloguing in Publication Data
Mounayer, Bonnie
    The back shop book
    1 Man. Back. Care
    I. Title   II. Wynn-Williams, Susan
    617'.56

    ISBN 0–356–17139–6

Macdonald & Co. (Publishers) Ltd
66–73 Shoe Lane
Holborn
London EC4P 4AB

Photoset in Helvetica by 🖝 Tek Art Ltd

Printed and bound in Great Britain by
Hazell, Watson & Viney Ltd
Aylesbury, Bucks

CONTENTS

PREFACE

'The essence of education is the education of the body.'

Benjamin Disraeli, 1804–1881

This book is the result of the many discerning questions and ideas put to us by customers visiting the Back Shop. We believe there is an obligation to respond to the needs of our customers, and so in this book, we aim to give them the information they seek for themselves and their families in an easy fashion without losing track in the complexity of the subject.

Many excellent books have been written by experts on the complicated subject of the back. Many questions are answered in them, but often they are highly technical. Medical words can be bewildering, confusing, lengthy or just vague, as well as biased by individual training. Orthodox medicine still tends to retain an air of mystery, with treatments recommended but not explained. When asked, practitioners may give evasive answers or not have the time to give advice.

In 1984 the Back Shop opened in London's West End close to Harley Street. It sells a wide range of products gathered from all over the world so that back pain sufferers can find the help they need under one roof. The idea behind the Back Shop is not new. Back shops have existed in the United States of America for some time. In the United Kingdom, we felt the concept of the Back Shop should be to provide informed professional expertise together with the widest possible range of products. This book is part of that exercise. We have purposely repeated ourselves to stress the importance of certain immutable precepts – anatomy, movement, mobility, posture, and most important of all, self-help.

Education is the cornerstone on which the future of the Back Shop rests. It is essential that we continue to pursue new discoveries and ideas from different cultures around the world. Modern technological advancements are important but we should not forget the ancient remedies which often provide immediate relief from back pain.

This book is for the general public to read and to put its recommendations into practice so they can prevent back pain. A moment's thoughtlessness can have devastating long-term effects. As well as causing physical and emotional discomfort, it is also expensive, both for individuals and their families, in treatment and loss of earnings, and nationally in sickness payment benefits.

Your back is meant to last a lifetime – look after it by using this book.

Bonnie Mounayer and Susie Wynn-Williams
1989

ACKNOWLEDGMENTS

This book would not have been possible without the enormous help of Marie O'Flaherty, who has coordinated the text, helped to select the quotations, organised the word-processing and bullied us to keep on schedule with a nurse's kind tolerance and incisive input. With the assistance of Romie Lamah, who did the typing, Anne Cooksey who read the proof having been a back school participant, Karen Addenbrooke and Dr Alan Bravermann, who kindly found time to cast a medical eye over the text, Valerie Pate who contributed patience and common sense, Karen Harper and Karen Rickman, the nursing staff in the shop, and most importantly, Judith Rowbotham PhD who cast an expert eye over the final text.

We would also like to thank illustrator Shaun Williams, Jayne Booth our editor, Harriet Griffey and Cécile Landau who encouraged us in the early stages, Aquarius, John Farbon Marketing Ltd, Walter Brearley, Scan Q Ltd, Spinal Publications, Bolton Stirland International, Scan-Sit, BMA Ergonomic, Bay Jacobsen, MeDesign Ltd, Partners, Putnam's Back Care Systems, Spenco Medical UK Ltd, Spencer (Banbury) Ltd, Ergoform, and Spine Seat Co.

Finally and most important, we thank our husbands for their tolerance and understanding.

INTRODUCTION

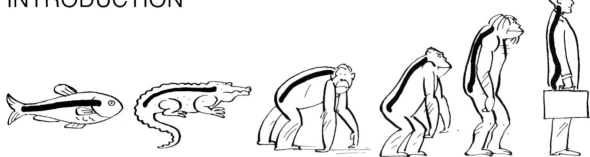

Human beings are designed to be very physical creatures and human performance relies on a good back: one free from pain, spasm, aches and tension. Yet for the population of the Western world, the main affliction of the twentieth century is back pain.

Our pre-historic ancestors walked miles as they hunted, climbed trees and were generally extremely active. Squatting was the position of choice for rest, and manual labour gave freedom from back pain. We evolved out of a jungle environment; children born today have the same physical structure as pre-historic man. In remote parts of the world, primitive peoples have very few instances of back pain. However, 'Homo Sedens' in the West has carefully brought about his own physical ruin. What has he done to cause so much discomfort and pain? He has failed to adapt to the changes brought about by advanced technology and improvements in the workplace. At the same time he has failed to maintain good back mobility in every day life.

The back is never still. Even breathing causes it to move as the rib cage expands and contracts, and it runs many risks in everyday life. In the garden, driving the car, playing a sport or turning on the bath tap, lifting or stretching, standing or sitting for long periods – hazards are everywhere for the back. When problems do occur they do not always disappear overnight. However 75 per cent recover in a week and 90 per cent within a month.

It is possible to relieve an acute attack quickly. Everyone, not only back sufferers, can benefit from this book, but you must be prepared to work at understanding the anatomy of the back, know how to avoid straining the muscles and joints by learning to lift correctly, and know how to cope with an acute attack of back pain. Determine for yourself:

- The common causes of backache.
- How you can relieve an acute back pain by simple home treatment.
- How you can organise a daily programme which is specific for your needs.
- How you can learn techniques and tips which will help your back and stop recurrences.
- How with simple home measures you can save hours of painful sitting in a doctor's surgery or a hospital treatment room.

If you have a problem and pain which persists beyond a reasonable time, you may be in the important minority who really need medical or surgical help. If anything your doctor says conflicts with the advice given in this book, always follow your doctor's instructions as he will be taking the individual characteristics of your back problem into account.

With 88,000 people a day off work in the United Kingdom and 4 out of 5 people every day seeing their doctor or other practitioners as a result of bad backs, it is vital to do something NOW.

Note and warning

If you feel any strain or pain on attempting any of the exercises in this book or if you are under medical supervision for back trouble, only follow the exercises subject to the advice of the doctor or other registered and qualified medical practitioners.

How to use this book

This book is designed for easy reference covering every aspect of back health and care. The entries are arranged alphabetically, with cross references which are printed in **bold italic** throughout.

At the back of the book there is a comprehensive reference section with addresses of useful organisations and practitioners, and suggestions for further reading with addresses of helpful bookshops.

THE SEVEN STAGES OF LIFE

The baby – 0 to 5

The seeds of back trouble may be sown early in life. At birth, the thorax, sacrum and coccyx remain curved in the same direction. These are the primary curves. The neck and then the lower back develop curves in the opposite direction to the primary curves as the child learns to control its head. These are called secondary curves.

Before a baby sits or walks, he or she should crawl along on all fours. This action teaches the baby to control its head and strengthen the neck muscles, which act like guy ropes to lift the head up so the secondary curve is formed in the neck region. The advantage of the curves is that the weight of the body, including the head, is balanced so that keeping upright is less tiring. The baby and growing toddler have a natural degree of balance and coordination of movement, so babies should not be encouraged into a sitting position before they can sit by themselves, and high chairs should not be abandoned too early.

The child – 5 to 12

By the age of 5 or 6 a child may spend several hours each day bent over a work table or school desk, sitting on flat, straight hard chairs which may be at incorrect levels. Children should not be put on adult chairs unless they have a footstool or until their feet can touch the floor, otherwise bad posture will be the result. Poor slumped posture produces a long-term strain on the soft bones, tendons and muscles of the growing back. Poorly designed furniture imposes symptoms on the backs of children at a critical time in their lives. During this period, when they are growing, it is vital that posture, especially the sitting posture, is corrected and watched continually, so school furniture is therefore very important and children should not remain sedentary but exercise frequently.

The teenager – 13 to 19

During adolescence the back is extremely vulnerable as it is growing and the strength of the muscles is not always adequate for all the activities enjoyed by this age group. Often rigorous sports programmes are undertaken, heavy school books and school bags are carried, and seating at schools and colleges is unsuitable. Crookedness or severe slouched shoulders and a round slumped back can result. Sometimes the vogue in current footwear – high or wedge heels, trainers – can cause an unbalanced posture, prevent correct gait and lead to flat feet. Teenagers should be encouraged both by their parents
and their teachers to think about their posture. The use of a mirror can be the best way to show them how they use their backs. If good habits for the back are started early in life it will pay dividends in the future.

The young adult – 20s to 30s

Whether carving out a career or having a family, back problems arise during this busy time. An accident, occupational hazards or pregnancy may be the cause of back trouble. Activities on the ski slopes, the rugby field, while playing tennis and squash or riding and fishing can all lead to strain and accidents to the back. Current fashion trends or an unsuitable car may also be the initial cause of backache. The hazards of smoking, drinking, working with computers or a military career may all lead to back problems. However, the incidence of back pain are low during this stage as the body should be at its physical peak.

The adult – 30s to 50s

The highest incidence of back trouble occurs in this age group, research showing that women are slightly more affected than men. Bringing up a family, with all the lifting and carrying of small children, shopping and general housework, can quickly lead to back problems. Regular exercise, rest and sleep, along with correct lifting and carrying techniques, will go a long way to preventing and alleviating backache.

Postural back pain is a common occurrence in a number of professions. Standing for a long time, sitting at a desk for long periods, carrying and lifting heavy weights without considering the stress and strain experienced by the back, can all lead to problems – office workers, surgeons, nurses, VDU operators, miners, construction workers, farmers and hairdressers are just some of the many people at risk. To avoid the hazards of everyday working life it is vital to plan the furniture for the home and workplace ergonomically.

Middle age – 50s to 70s

This time of life is now regarded as middle age, due to the increase in the elderly population. With the family grown up, there is more time to maintain a healthy back and develop good postural habits based on past experience. However, as we get older, degenerative joint disease will arise. The structures of the back will show signs of wear and tear. The muscles and ligaments become less elastic, so it is vitally important to take regular exercise and keep the back as supple as possible. Walking, swimming, ballroom dancing, bowling and golf are all enjoyable ways of keeping fit and supple. Care should also be taken to watch and control any increase in weight. Hormone replacement therapy may be used for women, after thorough investigation, to help avoid osteoporosis during and after menopause. Now is the time when suitable furniture which supports the back is well worth considering and may be more readily within the financial budget.

The elderly – 70+

In old age many people complain of aches and stiffness but not pain in the back. During this period the gristly discs between the bones of the back lose height by chemical dehydration, shrinkage occurs and the back can become physically bowed. The slippery surfaces of joints may roughen, and grating may be felt and even heard. However, by maintaining an active lifestyle and a good postural balance, backache can be minimal.

Keeping warm is vital to maintain good circulation and help is available through the social services if housework, lifting or driving become impossible. But sitting in front of the television set all day will not help – rest in excess can lead to 'rust'. Walking, swimming, bowls and gardening are all enjoyable pursuits for this group, providing energy levels are good. If there are signs of mental depression resulting in backache, due perhaps to loneliness or bereavement, joining a simple exercise class or group therapy may help to stop relegation to the dust heap, and perhaps increase the life span and enjoyment of good health.

ABDOMINAL MUSCLES

The abdomen is the area of the body between the diaphragm and the pelvis, and it is extremely important to have excellent tone in the abdominal **muscles** in order that the back can work efficiently. The muscles help stabilise the trunk and lower back or **lumbar region**, and play an essential role in the **pelvic tilt**.

The abdominal muscles are in three layers and are designed to act like a corset, supporting the trunk and balancing the flexible movements of the back. Since most of us spend too much time sitting every day, these muscles become lax and flabby and a bulging tummy is the result. A curved, bowed back and round shoulders will also develop, with the result that low back pain and a stiff neck frequently follow. Weak abdominal muscles may also result in a hernia or, in women, a prolapse of the uterus.

Strong firm abdominal wall muscles stop the internal organs such as the stomach and the intestines sagging forwards, prevent back strain and enable easy **lifting** movements. The natural increase of pressure in the abdominal cavity when you lift helps the mechanical load on the back.

Abdominal or 'tummy tightener' exercises

Perhaps most important of these exercises for the back is the **pelvic tilt**. To get down on the floor for these exercises, start by kneeling down. Then sit on your haunches. Put one hand on the floor at the side, followed by the other, lower yourself gently on to your bottom and stretch your legs out in front of you, placing one hand on either side for balance. Bend your knees and gently lower your back down to the floor.

Pelvic tilt

Lie on your back with your knees bent at a comfortable angle of about 45 degrees, knees slightly apart and your feet on the floor. Support your head and neck with a pillow and place your arms loosely by your sides.

Gently pull in your tummy muscles and squeeze your buttocks, flattening and pressing your lower back and waist against the floor. Don't arch the back or hold your breath. Spread one hand on your tummy to feel the contraction, hold for a count of five, then release slowly and rest for a count of five. Repeat five times, then gradually work up to ten repetitions. Try this exercise for a month if you want to see a difference.

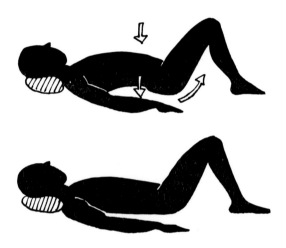

When you have perfected pelvic tilt lying down, practise it sitting and standing to strengthen your abdominal muscles.

Curling up

Lie on your back with your knees bent, and flatten the small of your back against the floor, as for pelvic tilt, keeping the chin tucked in.

Curl your head and shoulders forwards up off the floor, looking straight ahead. Slide your hands along your thighs, reaching forwards with your hands to touch the points of your knees with your fingertips. Hold for a count of five and then uncurl slowly, controlling the back, head and shoulders, to the starting position. Relax for a count of five. Repeat five times. Only curl as high as is comfortable. You should feel no tension in the neck or upper back – make the tummy muscles do the work.

NOTE AND WARNING: It is important not to drop your head suddenly as it will jar the upper back.

Progression exercise

Lie on your back with your knees bent, as for the pelvic tilt. Pull in the tummy. Raise one knee towards the chest until the hip is at a 90 degree angle. Lift the other knee to meet the first. Hold for a count of five. Return the feet to the floor. Repeat ten times. As a further progression, lower one leg first and slide it along the floor until extended. Bring it back up to meet the other leg. Hold for a count of five. Repeat with the other leg. Do this ten times.

NOTE AND WARNING: 'Sit up' exercises should NEVER be performed until you have good, strong abdominal muscles.

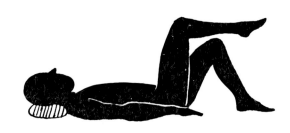

Progression exercise

ABNORMAL BACK

Some people may be born with an abnormal back or disability. This may be as a result of genes in the family, i.e. an inherited abnormality, or it can be caused by disease, an accident during pregnancy or childbirth. It is advisable to consult a doctor if there are any unusual signs present.

ABSCESS

Bacterial infection can cause an abscess around a **vertebra** or **disc**, but it is rare. Local tenderness and muscle spasm will develop. There will be a general feeling of being unwell, and perhaps a subsequent fever. Medical advice is necessary and antibiotics or injections may be given to destroy the bacteria.

ACTIVITY

When you are active you expend and exert energy. However activity is not the same as exercise. Activities such as sport, digging the garden, housework and driving should not be confused with regular specific exercises for mobilising and strengthening the back.

ACUPRESSURE

This is based on the same principle as **acupuncture**. The fingers or knuckles are pressed on the traditional acupuncture points to adjust the energy flow. Chinese and Japanese methods, for example **shiatsu**, are also used to stimulate tender points.

ACUPUNCTURE

The word acupuncture comes from two Latin words, *acus* meaning needles and *pungere* meaning to sting. Acupuncture involves the use of needles which are placed in the body at specific points.

Acupuncture comes from ancient China and is based on texts which are thousands of years old. It has gradually developed in the last 4,000–6,000 years throughout China, Tibet and northern India, finally reaching the Western world comparatively recently. Today there are two different styles of acupuncture; traditional acupuncture and scientific acupuncture.

Traditional acupuncture

This is based on Chinese medicine. The basic theory of traditional acupuncture is that a person's state of health is thought to depend on the balance between positive and negative forces – yin and yang – within the body. If these forces are in balance there is a free flow of energy – chi or qi – throughout the body; if there is an imbalance then the energy flow is impeded and problems will occur. Energy flows along 12 pairs of channels or pathways – the meridians – which run up and down the body.

In determining the pattern of disharmony or disease, the acupuncturist needs a detailed understanding of the patient's lifestyle. To reach a diagnosis involves questions, observation, examination of the appearance of the tongue and feeling the six pulses on each wrist corresponding to the 12 meridians. The rhythm and quality of the pulse indicates the balance of energy, and the tongue, through its shape, colour, movement and coating, shows the progression and degree of illness.

Scientific acupuncture

Scientific acupuncture is based on the theory that acupuncture can be used to stimulate the nervous system and therefore help to relieve pain. Scientists know that acupuncture causes the release of morphine-like substances called endorphins, which act as the body's own pain-killers.

Doctors, physiotherapists and nurses now practise acupuncture for the relief of pain in the back and for joint problems after they have established a conventional medical diagnosis.

Treatment

Acupuncture is applied most commonly with clean disposable stainless steel needles. The traditional acupuncturist will select points along the appropriate meridians. The needles are inserted at these specific points, in order to stimulate or curb the energy flow. The insertion of the needles is usually painless, or there may be a sharp stinging sensation for a second or two.

In acupuncture for the relief of pain, the medical practitioner will select points on the basis of the nerve supply; these correspond very much to the same points as in traditional acupuncture. The needles are left in position for anything from a few seconds to 15 or 30 minutes. During the treatment, the acupuncturist may adjust the needles by rotating them slightly.

Acupuncture treats the whole person, both in the physical and mental context. A feeling of relaxation can ensue after acupuncture and the symptoms may be relieved quite quickly: however some conditions can be aggravated, so it is wise to check with your doctor first and seek out a registered qualified practitioner whose address can be found by using the Where to Get Help and Suggested Further Reading sections at the end of this book.

ACUTE BACK

An acute back is when there is a sudden onset of inflammation and pain which is of brief duration. This is a crisis, which may be caused by a fall, a wrench, a strain, an activity, or something very trivial such as turning on the bath tap. It also may be due to heat, cold or an invasion of bacteria. An acute back comes on suddenly; immediate treatment is necessary.

There will be the following signs:

- *Pain*.
- Limitation of movement.
- Swelling.
- Protective muscle *spasm*.

What to do

- Stop what you are doing IMMEDIATELY and think what to do next. A minor injury or twinge can be turned into a more severe one if you continue with the activity that may be causing it. Telephone the doctor at once if you are worried and need medical advice.
- Lie down on a firm surface. Go to bed if it is supportive and if you can get there (see *beds*.) If not, lie on the floor, supported where possible with pillows. A light mattress or a piece of foam will soften the hardness of the floor.
- *Rest* for 24 hours in a lying position so the back no longer has to carry the weight of the body. The back cannot be rested by sitting down. Relax and try not to be apprehensive. You may need bed rest for two to three days. (See *positions*, *relaxation*.)

- Crawl on all fours to go to the bathroom and lavatory, getting in and out of bed carefully. When using the lavatory do not bend forwards. Avoid constipation, which will cause more pain, by eating plenty of fruit and roughage. Use a bedpan, bottle or bucket if the pain is so severe you cannot get out of bed. (See *toilets*.)
- Use heat or cold therapy, according to your tolerance and preference, for no longer than 15 minutes, three or four times a day. A hot water bottle, a Spenco Hot Wrap, an electric heating pad or infra-red lamp should give a gentle warmth only. Ice, a Spenco Cold Wrap or cold towels will also assist the circulation and relieve pain. (See *cold therapy*, *heat therapy*.)
  NOTE: If there is no skin sensation on touching the back, avoid using heat or cold therapy.
- Take *painkillers* such as *aspirin* or paracetamol which act as *anti-inflammatory* medication. Homeopathic remedies such as arnica or rhuta will also help relieve the inflammation.
- Wear a *support* or *corset* if your muscles are weak. Keep a *collar* and corset handy in case of an emergency until you can get to bed and rest. A simple lumbar belt such as the *Flexfit* is ideal.
- Start gentle movements gradually, once the peak of the pain has passed, to prevent stiffness and more pain. Exercises to correct *pelvic tilt* are extremely important and should be done first.
- A good *position* to relieve pain is to elevate the legs on to a chair or stool so that the hips and knees are at a 90 degree angle. The use of self *traction* with the *Trapeze* is beneficial if it is available.
- Have *showers*, not a *bath*, allowing the water to stimulate the circulation in the back.
- Give the back time to get better, and avoid starting manual work until the muscles have good *tone*. Don't carry or lift anything until you are better (see *carrying* and *lifting*.)
- If it hurts – DON'T DO IT.

ADHESIONS

When one adjacent surface sticks to another it is known as an adhesion. A sticky fluid is formed at the site of an inflammation causing the tissues, for example the muscles or ligaments in the back, to stick to each other. This sticky fluid becomes thickened, and fibrous tissue will form. Adhesions in the back can cause painful movement and *stiffness* will occur as a result. (See *fibrositis*.)

Adhesions can be broken down by a qualified registered practitioner, for example a chartered *physiotherapist*, an *osteopath* or a *chiropractor*. You will hear them use the word adhesions frequently, and they will employ *electrotherapy* as well as their fingers during treatment. (See *massage*.)

ADJUSTMENT

This is a term used by some manipulators to explain that they are putting something back in its place so that it is in normal working order. (See *manipulation*.)

ADVICE

Whenever you are in doubt about your back you should seek medical advice. An opinion will be given as to future action, in consultation with an orthodox medical practitioner or a member of one of the alternative therapies. Remember a registered qualified practitioner will have passed exams of the recognised body of medicine and may have many years' experience. Beware of 'cowboys' who set themselves up in practice after maybe a mere six-week correspondence course. And if you should listen to other people's advice, only follow it if it proves to be of help to you too.

The Where to Get Help section at the back of this book lists some of the addresses to enable you to find a practitioner.

AEROBICS

This is any exercise which involves pushing up the heart rate. The longer the exercise is performed and the faster it is done, the greater the endurance that will be achieved. The function of the heart, lungs and blood vessels are improved by aerobics, optimising the body's utilisation of oxygen. Aerobics is not necessarily jogging and fast sequences to music in dance exercise classes, it can be walking or cleaning the car.

Aerobic exercise can lead to improved **posture** and better **balance** of the back, but care should be taken not to jar the spine by rigorous **jogging** on hard surfaces and by overdoing the exercises. Remember you can walk and swim aerobically.

AEROBICYCLES

These are computerised exercise bicycles for **warming up** on before a workout.

AGILITY

Agility is the ability to move quickly and change direction rapidly and smoothly while maintaining control of the back and body. Agility is essential for sports activities, especially contact sports such as rugby, basketball and squash, if back injuries and problems are to be prevented.

AGONY

Intense back pain can cause a lot of suffering, so if a person is in agony treat it like an **acute back** and seek medical advice.

AIDS FOR DAILY LIVING

See **useful products**.

AIR CONDITIONING

The change of temperature and the cool draughts that can arise with air conditioning cause back problems, especially if the vent is located near the back of your chair.

Move your desk at work away from any vents, as the lower back and neck are the most susceptible regions and you will thus avoid **lumbago** or an acute stiff neck.

The contrast of going from the heat outside into an air conditioned room in a hot climate can also cause problems. The muscles go into spasm with the temperature change, and any moisture on the skin can become cold and damp resulting in **trigger points**. Check the back of your shirt or blouse for dampness – it is worth keeping a dry clean one in the office so you can change it immediately if it is at all wet. (See **backache**.)

AIR TRAVEL

What to do

- It is often helpful for back pain sufferers when travelling by aeroplane to use a lumbar roll or a curved lumbar support in the small of the back. If you do not have one, there are always small pillows on board which can be obtained from the air hostess. (See **supports**.)
- If your head is not adequately supported and there is a gap behind the neck, then a small cervical **pillow** or an inflatable curved neck support will help. (See **collars**.)
- Tall people have trouble with inadequate leg room in planes. Whenever possible obtain one of the seats on the aisle, near the emergency exit or next to the partitions and the cinema screen, where there is more leg room.
- If you have back problems do not hesitate to make a request for suitable seating at the check-in desk prior to boarding the aircraft.

- Short people whose feet do not touch the floor should place a small piece of luggage or a pile of magazines on the floor to prop up their feet, if the crew cannot provide a foot rest.
- A frequent walk up and down the aisle to maintain mobility is advisable, especially on long flights. (See **walking**.)
- A *corset* or neck collar should be worn for air travel if there are any painful back or neck symptoms.
- In-flight luggage should be carried by a porter or put on a trolley. (See **carrying** and **lifting**.)
- If you are receiving medical treatment for back pain, your medical practitioner can write a letter to the airport authorities, who are usually extremely helpful in providing facilities such as a wheelchair.

- If you have an **acute back** it is not wise to fly.

ALCOHOL

Excess alcohol intake should be avoided, as it affects the body tissues. A pain can result in the back if internal organs become inflamed due to too much alcohol. It also disturbs the balance of the body, which can lead to accidents, injuries and back strain.

ALEXANDER TECHNIQUE

This technique was developed by Matthias Alexander, an actor, who was born in Tasmania in

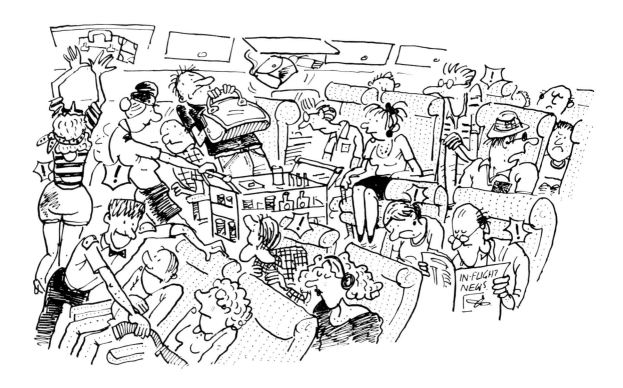

1869. It is a method which teaches about good **posture** and **relaxation**, based on the knowledge that habitually incorrect posture, movement and tension may have an adverse effect on the body as a whole. Practitioners teach you through gentle manual guidance how to support and balance your body, and how to relax in everyday life so that mental attitudes and emotional equilibrium do not become problems. Lessons are on an individual basis.

The Alexander Technique is very useful in helping back pain due to postural defects and in preventing recurrence of old bad habits which may cause an acute episode. However, the Alexander Technique alone will not cure an **acute bad back**. The address of the organisation can be found in the Where To Get Help section at the end of the book.

ALTERNATIVE MEDICINE

See **complementary medicine**.

ANAEROBIC EXERCISE

Anaerobic exercise is very hard and fast exercise over a short time, after which rest is needed, with fairly heavy breathing control, in order to pay back the oxygen deficit that has occurred in the muscles during the exercise; for example, in sprinting and basketball. The muscles that support the back and the abdominal muscles should be in very good condition if this form of exercise is undertaken, as agility and balance are essential.

ANALGESICS

Analgesia means relief of pain, so analgesics are drugs designed to stop pain. If you are unable to sleep and are in severe pain, strong analgesics may be given by the doctor for a few days. (See **aspirin, drugs, painkillers**.)
NOTE: Analgesics do not affect the cause of the pain, just relieve the symptoms.

ANATOMY OF THE BACK

The study of the form and arrangement of the various structures which make up the body is called anatomy.

The design of the back has evolved to its present form over millions of years. Mechanically, it connects the head, shoulder girdle, pelvic girdle and legs, providing suspension for the arms and ribcage.

The functions of the back are:

- To provide the strong central support for the upright **posture** of the human body. This posture enables you to use your arms and hands for everyday manual skills, both at work and play.
- To protect the **spinal cord** and nerve roots.
- To allow flexibility for a range of movements, permitting you to bend, twist, turn, squat, lift, push and pull without falling over.

The anatomy of the back shows a structure of blocks of small bones, the **vertebrae**, stacked on top of each other like a child's building bricks. There are 33 vertebrae, some of which are fused, so that there are only 24 individual bones. The bones are divided into regions:

- **Cervical region** or **neck**   7 vertebrae
- **Thoracic region** or chest   12 vertebrae
- **Lumbar region** or lower   5 vertebrae
  back
- Sacral region or **sacrum** 5 fused vertebrae
- Coccygeal region,   4 fused vertebrae
  coccyx or tail

These specific areas are all part of the total structure of the back and are interdependent, so if something happens in the neck region it will nearly always effect some other region of the back. (See **curves**.)

At the back of each individual vertebrae are two small **joints**, the facet joints, which slide or glide against each other, controlling the range and direction of movement and providing stability. In between each bone and the next are structures acting like shock absorbing cushions, called intervertebral **discs**. These discs prevent

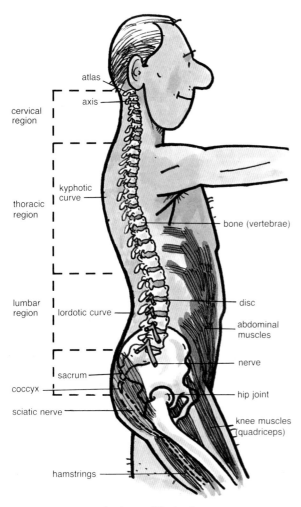

atlas
axis
cervical region
kyphotic curve
thoracic region
bone (vertebrae)
lumbar region
lordotic curve
disc
abdominal muscles
nerve
sacrum
coccyx
hip joint
sciatic nerve
knee muscles (quadriceps)
hamstrings

Anatomy of the back

the bones grating or rubbing against each other and allow flexibility of the back.

The bones are held together by strong supporting tough fibrous bands of tissue, called **ligaments**, which are slightly elastic. They stabilise the back by controlling and guiding the movements which are performed by **muscles**. The muscles play a supporting, protective and balancing role so that the back is able to function correctly.

The vital spinal cord of nerves lies in the spinal canal, a hole running through the middle of each vertebra. It runs up the centre of the column formed by the backbone, relaying and conducting messages to the brain and all parts of the body. (See **nervous system**.)

ANGER

Anger can cause muscular tightness and tension in the back. Learn to identify this emotion. Jerky tense movements while you tell your nearest and dearest to shut up, or bottling up feelings so that you sit rigidly in a chair and keep your thoughts enclosed behind a tightly shut mouth, will only lead to headaches, stiffness in the neck and pain in the back.

What to do

- Learn to identify your **emotions** when you are angry, so that you maintain control and do not have jerky movements or **tension** in the back muscles.
- Let your anger out. You do not have to shout and get in a rage with people. You want to keep your friends! Have a good yell or shout or even cry – perhaps somewhere where no one can hear you.
- Write a letter to the person to vent your anger – you will probably end by tearing it up.
- Take some form of physical activity; for example, walk off your anger. (See **walking**.)
- If you are very competitive and lose your temper easily, try to **relax** more and learn to concentrate on deep **breathing** as an alternative.
- Regular **massage** of the back often helps this form of tension.
- Seek the guidance of a good counsellor.

ANGLES

See **chairs** and **hips**.

ANIMALS

Certain animals suffer from bad backs. The force of gravity is a problem for all animals and the gravitational force on upright or vertical animals has proved to be less than on those in the horizontal position, i.e. those that stand on all fours.

In four-legged animals, the backbone functions like a suspension bridge, supported by the four legs acting as pillars. Man has only two pillars, as the arms are up in the air, so the support comes from the muscles fore and aft acting like the guy ropes of a tent.

Horses, especially racehorses, and dogs such as dachshunds with long backs are especially susceptible to pain in the back, and vets now work in conjunction with physical therapists to make sure that the damaged muscles are treated as quickly as possible so that the animal has the strength to overcome gravity and avoid further muscular injuries and back problems. Swimming is found to be a great benefit to animals.

ANKLE

The joint which connects the lower leg with the foot. The ankle must be mobile and stable as weak ankles can cause poor **posture** of the back in standing and walking, which in turn may lead to back strain. Also if the ankles are weak, **balance** will be poor, resulting in back injuries when playing a sport or dancing.

A useful exercise to mobilise the ankles is to rotate both ankles by moving them frequently in a clockwise and anti-clockwise direction during the day. This is especially beneficial if you are confined to bed.

ANKYLOSING SPONDYLITIS

This term comes from two Greek words. Spondylitis is derived from the Greek word for vertebra, *spondylos*, while *itis* means **inflammation**. So it means inflammation of the vertebrae. As the inflammation subsides, bone forms from both sides of the joint, enclosing it completely during the healing process. The bony formation results in fusion and causes immobility. This fixation or stiffness is ankylosis.

Therefore, ankylosing spondylitis is an arthritic condition of the vertebral joints of the back (see **arthritis**). It mainly affects young adults, the predominance being amongst young men in their 20s and 30s. It can also affect the tissues and the joints of the limbs. The cause is unknown.

If you think you have ankylosing spondylitis, see the doctor immediately. Treatment is usually straightforward and should be started as soon as possible to prevent long-term loss of movement and deformity. (See Where to Get Help.)

ANNULUS

The outer layer of a **disc** is termed the annulus.

ANOREXIA

A nervous condition in teenagers and young adults, manifested in an obsessive desire to slim. It can lead to a severe loss of weight, with the result that the muscles of the back and the abdomen can become wasted. There is a subsequent lack of energy, resulting in back strain and pain.

ANTENATAL

Back problems can arise in this period before **childbirth**. *(See **pregnancy**.)*

ANTI-DEPRESSANTS

These drugs may be prescribed by the doctor to prevent the depression which can arise as a result of a chronic bad back or if emotional problems have heightened the pain.
NOTE: They do not affect the cause of the pain but just relieve the symptoms.

ANTI-INFLAMMATORY

Anti-inflammatory drugs are given to relieve back

pain on the assumption that the back pain is due to **inflammation** in the tissues. They can have side effects such as drowsiness or gastric upset, so follow the doctor's prescription carefully.
NOTE: They do not affect the cause of the pain but just relieve the symptoms.

ANXIETY

'When you're lying awake with a dismal headache,
And repose is taboo'd by anxiety,
I conceive you may use
Any language you choose
To indulge in without impropriety.'
W.S. Gilbert, 1836-1911

Everyone is anxious sometimes and this may prevent sleep, interfere with work and cause physical symptoms such as headaches, tension and muscle spasm. If you have chronic back pain you may become extremely anxious and worried, which will lead to further stress, and in some cases panic.

What to do

* Try and learn to recognise this **emotion**.
* Learn **breathing** and **relaxation** techniques.
* Have counselling.

See **stress** and the Suggested Further Reading section at the end of the book.

'A trouble shared is a trouble halved.'

ARCHING

Like all animals, especially cats and dogs, a human being needs to arch and stretch the back; this is also called **extension**. Specific arching **exercises** may be given to relieve low back **pain**. (See **mobilising**.)

ARMCHAIRS

See **chairs**.

ARMS

Movements of the back can cause pain in the upper limbs of the body. This may be due to:

* Incorrect **lifting** and **carrying**, which will result in pain in the arms if the back is not used correctly.
* Violent jerking of the **neck**; this may cause pain in the shoulders and upper arms, which can radiate down to the hands and fingers.
* Manual activities such as **decorating** or window cleaning.

It is extremely important to have the arms in the correct **position** when performing activities and exercises, at work, at play, or during sleep. For example, there is more demand on the abdominal muscles with the hands placed behind the head or elevated at full stretch in the air.

ARTHRITIS

The term arthritis is frequently misused by the general public. The Greek word *arthron* means joint, while *itis* means inflammation, so it is an **inflammation** in the **joints** resulting from injury, infection or from disease. The four most common types are:

* Osteoarthritis, correct name **osteoarthrosis**, is also sometimes called 'wear and tear' arthritis.
* **Rheumatoid arthritis**.
* **Gout**.
* **Ankylosing spondylitis**.

Most kinds of arthritis can be treated and improve with treatment.

ARTHROGRAPHY

This is a technique used to determine whether pain is caused by **inflammation** or **osteo-arthrosis** in the **joints**. A local injection is given to anaesthetise the area and a small amount of dye is injected which shows up on an X-ray, allowing the specialist to verify the position of the joint.

ARTIFICIAL JOINTS

Joint replacement is not commonly used in the back, due to its extreme complexity and the position of the nervous system. However, it is extremely important to re-educate the back to align **balance** after a total hip replacement or the attachment of an artificial limb, so that walking does not cause problems.

ASPIRIN

This is a common **painkilling** and **anti-inflammatory** drug which helps cope with most aches and pains. Aspirin can be bought over the counter at the chemist and is often found in combination with other drugs in tablet or soluble form. Aspirin should be taken as instructed when the pain is acute, but it is not advisable to take it if you have any gastric upset or there are any signs of a stomach or duodenal ulcer.
NOTE: It does not affect the cause of the pain but just relieves the symptoms.

ASSESSMENT

An expression used by practitioners to describe the procedure carried out to establish what is wrong with the back. (See **examination**.)

ASTHMA

The wheezing, shortness of breath and over-breathing that occur in this condition cause tension in the back. The breathing mechanism which moves the back as the ribcage expands and contracts becomes stiff.

What to do

- See a qualified medical practitioner to obtain correct medication.
- Learn specialised **breathing** techniques.
- Have **relaxation** exercises.
- Obtain counselling.

ATLAS

The first of the **cervical** or **neck vertebrae**. The atlas vertebra largely consists of a socket into which the odontoid peg of the *axis* vertebra fits. The atlas allows nodding movements to take place between the skull and the axis. The atlas may be affected in **rheumatoid arthritis**.

AUTONOMIC NERVOUS SYSTEM

See **nervous system**.

AVULSION

See **fracture**.

AWARENESS

Be aware of your shape. Basically there are three main body shapes:

Ectomorphs

Ectomorphs tend to have long bones and a straight slender shape. They are naturally thin and never really put on weight no matter how much they eat; as a result they may often lack energy and their muscle tone may be poor.

Mesomorphs

Mesomorphs can be tall or short. This group are muscular and powerful. They have broad developed shoulders and slim hips. They are very active with plenty of energy and find it easy to exercise.

Endomorphs

Endomorphs are rounded and not very tall. They have small hands and feet but wide hips and usually heavy bodies, and can have weight problems.

AXIS

The second of the **neck** or **cervical vertebra**. The axis has a large projecting process, the odontoid peg, sticking up from its top surface. This peg rotates in the socket of the *atlas* vertebra forming a pivot **joint**, which allows turning of the head. The axis may be affected with the atlas in **rheumatoid arthritis**. (See **anatomy**.)

BABIES

Caring for a baby can produce several hazards for the back as you will frequently have to lift a baby in and out of a cot or pram. This is perhaps more of a risk for the mother whose *ligaments* have weakened during *pregnancy*.

What to do

- Always think how you are going to carry the baby and try not to upset the *balance* of your back by *carrying* the child on one hip.
- Carry the baby in a special back pack designed for babies or in a sling worn close to the chest, providing it is firm and the baby is not too heavy. This means you carry the baby near your centre of gravity and therefore minimise the risk of back problems.

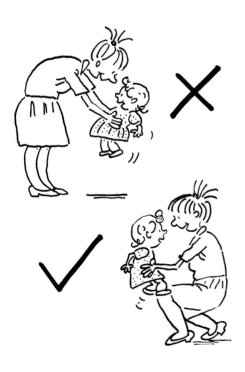

- Have a drop-sided cot to avoid bending over, and squat by *bending* your knees, keeping the feet close to the side of the cot. Lift the baby slowly, keeping the weight close to your chest. (See *squatting*, *lifting*.)
- If you have a carrycot for the baby, make sure it is placed in a position that is high enough to avoid bending or stooping when you pick it up. A table top, a bed or the top of a chest may be the best position for the cot.
- Always take the carrycot separately if you are taking the baby in the car as the weight of the baby in the cot will strain your back, unless there are two of you to carry it.
- When bathing the baby either kneel or squat, placing a special baby bath across the big bath so the height is more convenient for your back.
- Changing a baby is often best performed *kneeling* on the bed or the floor. If you have a piece of furniture at the right height, there is a special nappy changing unit to put on top so it is at the right level for your back.
- Prams and push chairs should have handles that enable you to push correctly. Choose a light pram that collapses easily for travelling.
- A father with a bad back should not use it as an excuse to avoid being involved with the baby, unless his back is acutely painful. Just adjust the height for all the baby activities as it is very rare that mothers and fathers are the same height. Grandparents too!

For the baby

- A thick nappy will provide cushioning and padding, protecting against any *jarring* or vibration of the growing back when the baby falls over in the early walking stages or against the bumping motion that sometimes occurs in sitting, often when one leg is tucked underneath and the baby is propelling itself with the other leg.

- Don't prop your baby up into a seated position until he or she can sit unaided and the muscles have strengthened by movement and crawling.
- Let the baby decide when it is ready to get up. Don't pull the baby up by the arms into a standing position until he can stand alone.
- Babies' *feet* should be left as free as possible as they are soft, easily pliable and can be distorted by tight boots, socks and all-in-one suits where the feet may not have a chance to straighten out and grow in a correct position. (See *shoes*.)
- Baby Walkers and baby bouncers can be dangerous since they often do not give adequate support and the vibrations can affect the growing back.

BACKACHE

Backache is almost as prevalent as the common cold, and it can be uncommonly painful. It is not a disease but a sign that something is wrong. An ache in the back can be prevented as the cause is usually mechanical.

Backache may be called many things. All these are popular general expressions:

- *Fibrositis*.
- *Lumbago*.
- *Arthritis*.
- Slipped *disc*.
- *Back strain*.
- *Muscle tear*.
- *Sciatica*.
- *Period* pain.

Causes of backache

- Poor *posture*.
- Inadequate weak *muscles*, sometimes caused by growing too fast.
- *Lifting* and *carrying* incorrectly.
- Carrying heavy weights constantly.
- An old sagging *bed*.
- Straight horizontal *chairs*.

- Driving a long way without a break (see *cars*).
- Wearing high-heel shoes (see *feet*).
- Stiffness from over-*exercise*.
- Chill (see *draughts* and *air conditioning*).
- *Period* pains.
- *Pregnancy*.
- *Depression*.
- *Anxiety* and *worry*.
- A fall or a jar on the back (see *jarring*).
- Overdoing it.
- Emotional tension and *stress*.
- *Kidney* trouble.

The lower back, since it is very mobile, is the most common site of backache, which can result from a simple action such as:

- Turning on a *bath* tap.
- Pulling a sheet off a *bed*.
- Tying a shoelace.
- Opening a window.
- Yawning, *coughing* or *sneezing*.

Loss of movement occurs to a varying degree, with an increase in pain when you attempt to move. Strain on the low back can affect the normal mobility of the joints, even altering the curvature (see *curves*) which puts an added strain on the *joints*, *muscles*, *ligaments* and *discs*.

Acute backache

This is when there is a sudden rapid onset of pain which may be sharp and intense, so you feel you are in agony and there is a loss of movement. It usually results from a slip, a fall, through coughing or some unaccustomed exercise. (See *acute back*.)

Recurrent backache

This is when episodes of pain appear in a routine fashion, usually as a result of performing similar movements in a regular pattern and in certain positions.

Chronic backache

This is when pain persists for several months. Movement may or may not be limited, and the pain may vary so that it is difficult to identify the cause and eliminate the backache. (See *chronic back*.)

How to avoid backache

- Use one *pillow* when sleeping, as high pillows strain the neck and shoulders.
- Sit up in a *chair*, making sure you are well supported, as sagging and slumping increases the strain on the neck and shoulders. (See *supports*, *useful products*.)
- *Stand* up well with an erect *posture* in a relaxed fashion, with your weight evenly distributed on both feet and correct *pelvic tilt*.
- Avoid increasing the lower back *curve* in the *lumbar region* when sitting and standing. (See *lordosis*.)
- Have a good *bed* with a supportive *mattress* and learn how to get in and out of bed correctly.
- Always bend your knees, not your back, when picking up and *lifting* objects, whether they are light or heavy.
- When *carrying*, balance the weight evenly on both sides.
- When *gardening*, kneel to weed, plant and sow seeds.
- Be fit not fat, as being overweight will cause *strain* on the *muscles* of the back.
- Never *exercise* unless you warm up first and cool down at the end of a routine, keeping an even body temperature all the time.

BACKFRIEND

A product from MeDesign which has been specially developed to support the whole back. (See *chairs*.)

BACK SCHOOL

The concept of back school was first conceived by a Swedish physiotherapist, Marianne Forsell in 1969. Back schools have since developed in the United States of America, Australia and the United Kingdom. Education and establishing new patterns of how to use the back are the basis of a back school. Classes are organised to teach back care and self help for the future prevention of back problems. Groups may number from six to fifteen people and classes will take place over a period of two to twelve weeks, according to the school. Every individual has a physical examination and a clinical assessment of the back.

The main subjects taught in back school are:

- Basic anatomy, physiology and the mechanics of the back.
- Postural advice on all positions.
- Correct lifting and handling techniques.
- Specific exercises for the muscles which support the back.
- What can go wrong with the back and how to avoid problems.
- How to cope with an acute painful back.
- How to choose furniture for the home and the workplace.
- Swimming and other activities.

Ask your doctor if there is one in your region or if the local hospital conducts a back school.

BACTERIA

A bacterial infection can occur in the back causing an *abscess* on the *vertebra*, but it is comparatively rare. Antibiotics will probably be prescribed by your doctor to combat the infection.

BADMINTON

This is a demanding *sport*. Wear good footwear to prevent *jarring* if you play on a composition surface rather than a sprung floor. Striking the shuttlecock in an off balance position strains the back joints, especially when **arching** the back for overhead shots.

BAGS

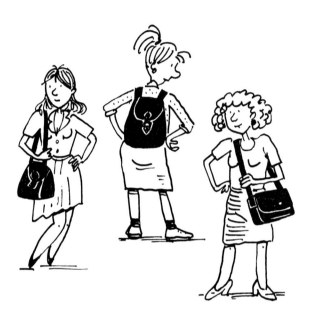

The best way to carry a bag is on the back because it distributes the weight evenly, lessening the chance of back or neck strain. If a backpack is not your style, the next best option is a shoulderbag slung diagonally across your body so that the weight is not concentrated in one area. Carrying a bag on one shoulder puts all the weight on one side of your body; if you have to use this method, put the bag on your non-dominant arm, i.e. if you are right handed, carry the bag on your left shoulder. This will protect the dominant arm from overuse, but no matter which method you choose keep the bag as light as possible to avoid undue muscle **strain**.

BALANCE

There has to be a balance between the back muscles and the **abdominal muscles** in order to preserve a good upright *posture* and avoid back problems. (See **biomechanics**, **muscles**.) You need good balance for all activities and sports to avoid **strains**, falls and other potential hazards.

Exercise to balance back and abdominal muscles

Position yourself on your hands and knees with the tummy pulled in and the correct **pelvic tilt**. The hands should be directly under the points of the shoulders and the knees should be hip-width apart.

Bring one knee in towards your nose, pointing the toe. Round the back and relax the neck and shoulders down towards the floor.

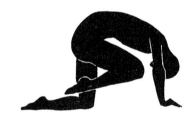

Finally, stretch the same leg up and back lifting it parallel to the floor and at the same time raising the head. Hold for five and relax. Repeat with the other leg.

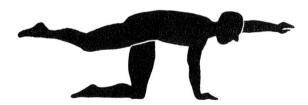

The sequence can be progressed for better balance by raising an alternate arm and leg.

NOTE: Make sure the movements flow throughout and don't jerk the leg up and back; your spine will not like it.

BALANS

This is the name – the Norwegian word for 'balance' – given to the seating which was created in Norway in the late 1970s. Credit for the original concept goes to Hans Christian Mengschoel, although four designers have been involved in the development. The first was a Norwegian, Peter Opsvik, a furniture designer, who as a result of meeting Dr Aage **Mandal** designed a seat with a forward tilt. Since Mandal advocated a chair with a seat that tilts 15 degrees forward, Opsvik incorporated this feature in his designs. Hans Christian Mengschoel found himself eating dinner while kneeling at a low coffee table and had the idea of inventing a kneeling stool or chair, since kneeling is natural and children often play in this position. He met Opsvik in 1978 and, with the encouragement of Addvin Rykken, a kneeling stool was produced, and the Balans seating is the result. (See **chairs**.)

BALLET DANCING

The back of a dancer requires agility and balance to perform the graceful, fine, precise movements of ballet. Any young person wishing to make a career in dancing should ensure that the back has no **congenital disorders**, no deformities such as **scoliosis**, nor has suffered any injury which might lead to arthritic changes and abnormality. (See **arthritis**.)

Dancers at all levels of ballet have to do a routine of exercises every day to remain at peak performance. It is hard work, with hours spent at the *barre* in order to strengthen and train the body, so careful checks by professional teachers and orthopaedic specialists while the back is growing may help the dancer prevent a bad back in the future. (See **orthopaedics**, as well as the section at the end of the book on Where To Get Help.)

BAR STOOLS

See **pubs**.

BASKETBALL

This popular **sport** is played in a forward **bending** position, with quick stretching motions to shoot a basket. The repetitive bounce of the ball with the quick **arching** and reaching movements can cause strain on the back, so it is important to warm up, exercise all muscle groups in the back and wear good supportive cushioned shoes when playing this sport.

BATHS

A warm, not a hot, bath can be a relaxing pain-relieving measure for muscle spasm in the back.

Tips

If you have back pain:

- Take care getting in and out of the bath. If you have acute back pain it might prove too strenuous for the first two days.
- Get someone else to turn on the taps if possible. Otherwise, take care turning on the taps, bend the knees and do not twist the back.
- Make sure there are no draughts in the bathroom.
- Have a warm towel. Wrap yourself in the bath towel rather than twisting to dry. Two or three small towels are preferable to one big one, so you can stand on one and use the other two for the rest of the body by looping them round your limbs.
- Try gentle **pelvic tilt** movement in the bath.
- A raised bath seat is a useful item of equipment for a very painful back or a chronic stiff back with limited movement. These are readily available in the shops.

- Cleaning the bath can be performed in a squatting position while in the bath but remember, a bit of dirt never hurt!

BAY JACOBSEN

See **beds**.

BEDDING

See **beds**.

BEDS

> 'O bed O bed Delicious bed
> That heaven on earth to a weary head.'
> Thomas Hood, 1799-1845

Beds are extremely important for the back since on average a third of your life is spent sleeping, regenerating the mind and the body. Maximum relaxation comes from the anatomically correct position so there are no painful signals or discomfort.

The base

This must be firm, not sagging or very springy. A wooden slatted base or the floor are ideal.

Firm-edge bases
These contain springs within a rigid frame. They are a good choice if you use the bed for seating as well. The wear and tear on the outer edge of the mattress will not be so great and with a firm base it will be easier to get up if you have a bad back.

Sprung edge bases
These have the springs on top of the frame so a greater area of comfort is available right to the edges of the base. They can be difficult to get out of if they are too springy, thus causing a strain on the back.

Unsprung bases
These are ideal for those who want a really firm bed. They are usually less expensive than sprung bases and vary from wooden slats to simple wooden bases covered in foam.

Getting in and out of bed

When getting into bed, sit on the side of the mattress, lower the body on to the elbow and shoulder, then bend up the knees until the feet can slide on to the bed and roll on to your back.

Reverse this process when getting out. Bend your knees up, roll on to your side keeping your knees together, then push up into a sitting position with your hand, allowing your legs to swing slowly down to the floor.

Always roll on to the least painful side when getting in and out of bed.

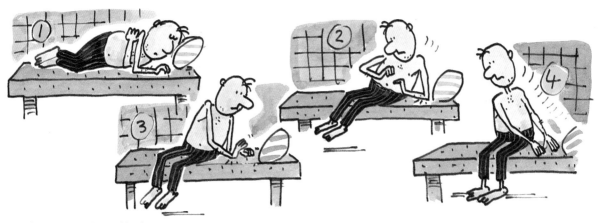

Getting in and out of bed

Double beds

Choose a double bed carefully. The minimum width is 5 ft but 5 ft 6 in or 6 ft is better. And don't be embarrassed about trying it out in the shop; partners differ in height and weight, and the amount of movement of the individual will vary during the night – it is estimated that we turn over between 70 and 100 times during the course of a night. Go shopping for a bed when you are both feeling fresh. If you're feeling at all tired, every bed will feel wonderful.

PARTNERS BEDS

The Partners range of beds was developed in 1983 by Marcus Bellati. The beds feature a comprehensive choice of specifications designed to take into account any relevant medical history, current back symptoms, overall weight distribution and any individual requirements such as height, weight, access and storage. Each bed is made to measure for the individual, using the best materials available in order to give comfort and durability.

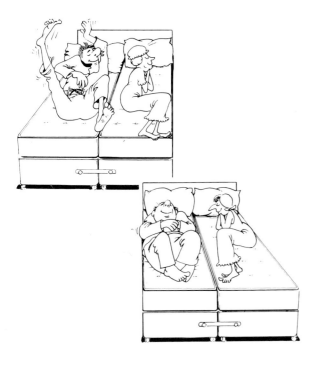

Useful hints when buying a bed

- Spend time trying out several different types of beds, for conformity to shape and with a firm but not a hard base. When assessing the degree of firmness you require, you should consider your height and weight.
- Have a mattress which supports the spine, but also allows the hips and shoulders to sink in when lying on your side.
- The height of the bed is important, so in order to establish what is comfortable, sit on the edge of the bed with the knees at a right angle. If you set the bed height slightly higher than the bend of the knees, it will help if you have back pain. It is recommended that the height should be adjustable within the range of 38 cm (15 in) to a minimum of 52 cm (20 in), taking into consideration the needs of the rest of the family if you are confined to bed and they have to look after you.
- When buying a double bed both people should try it. If one person gets off a double bed the other one should not feel any movement. Do not buy a double bed with a firm-edge base as your combined weight will depress the springs below the level of the firm edge, creating a trough.
- Find out which *position* is best for lying. If you lie on your back, try a pillow beneath your knees.
- Generally, heavier people need a firmer bed, so if your partner is 15 stone (95 kg) and you are only 8 stone (50 kg), you will need two singles linked at the base and zipped so each bed is suited to the individual and the lighter person will not fall towards the heavier one.

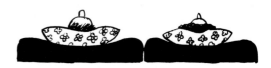

- A very firm mattress can be relieved by covering the bed with a layer of foam.
- For travelling or home use, a board can be used under a soft mattress to make it firmer.

Many hotels have a board available on request.

- Try a **waterbed**. They are supportive without exerting pressure on the hips and shoulders. A flotation mattress spreads the body weight evenly and you can have constant warmth with a heated waterbed.
- **Futons** are also worth considering as they save space and use the firm floor as a base.
- Adjustable beds are good for chronic back sufferers and help elderly people to be extremely comfortable.
- The recommended length for a bed is at least 188 cm (74 in) and preferably more to allow for greater comfort.
- A good bed lasts only for about 10 years, so if yours has reached this age it is time to throw it away and buy a new one, even if you think it is still comfortable.
- Do not buy a secondhand bed or accept a secondhand bed as a present.
- Do not be misled by labels such as 'orthopaedic' or 'firm'.
- Take advice from a medical practitioner or a good bed manufacturer.

Invest in a good bed. Your back will reap the dividends.

Bedding

Warm bedding is advisable and the shoulders and neck should be covered in order to avoid any draughts and consequent muscle spasm. (See **pillows**.)

WOOLREST SLEEPER

This product originated in New Zealand in 1979 and has been widely researched in Australia, America and the United Kingdom. The Woolrest Sleeper is made of pure wool, Kiwiwool, which is processed by Fleeciweave construction, so no use is made of adhesives, rubber or anything artificial which may aggravate the back. The relief of pressure and friction of this form of mattress topper which covers the entire sleeping area of a bed, protects vulnerable areas such as the shoulders, elbows, hips and knees, which are cushioned by the long thick fibres of Kiwiwool.

Research has shown that babies on this sort of lambswool bedding sleep more soundly, move less and are less likely to become uncovered, with a subsequent improvement in weight gain.

BAY JACOBSEN MATTRESS TOPPER

The Bay Jacobsen mattress overlay consists of layers of foam surrounding inner ducts filled with polystyrene granules. These granules help to maintain the body temperature so you stay warm and snug, at the right temperature and humidity.

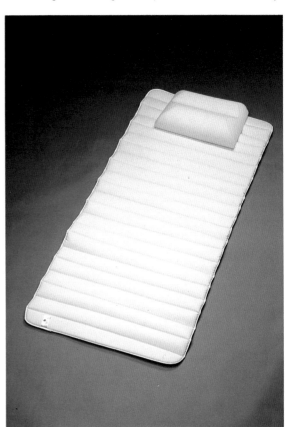

The Bay Jacobsen Mattress Topper

Bedmaking

Fitted sheets and duvets are a great help for a bad back as they make bedmaking easier.

Kneel down for tucking in sheets and put one

foot on the base for pulling off sheets. **Squatting** with the tummy braced is also a good way if you have strong thigh muscles.

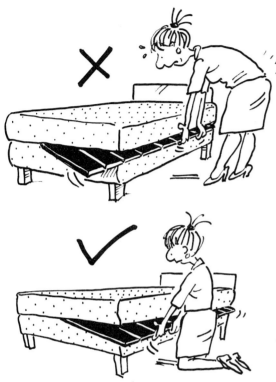

Making a bed (with a board)

Mattresses

A mattress should be firm so that the back has good support and does not sag or curve un-naturally – a two-layer mattress with 10–30 per cent compression in the 10–cm (4-inch) top layer, placed on a level non-yielding base, is the research recommendation. If a mattress is not firm enough, a bed board can be placed under-neath.

Conventional mattresses may be made of springs or old-fashioned horsehair, while a thin layer of foam placed on the floor is good if you have an **acute back** and you cannot get to bed. A **futon** or **waterbed** may also suit you. The optimum comfortable position is where the spine is an S-shape when viewed from the side and in a straight line when viewed from the back on a firm surface.

If a mattress is too hard a billiard-table effect causes discomfort of the hips and shoulders and distortion of the back: if it's too soft, worn out, and sagging, perhaps with a few broken springs, a hammock effect occurs which gives the spine no support.

There are various mattresses to choose from:

- Horsehair – the old-fashioned mattress stuffing.
- Spring-interior mattresses may have single open springs in fabric pockets or continuous coiled wires. The springs are sandwiched between layers of felt padding and topped by a layer of wool or synthetic fibres.
- Layers of foam are now used. They may be natural latex or a polyurethene mixture, and have the advantage of sometimes being non-allergic.
- Waterbeds are an alternative.
- Mattress toppers are available to soften hard mattresses.
- Sheepskin as a mattress overlay provides an effective back-warming surface.

To test a mattress
- Lie flat on the bed and slide the hand into the small of the back. If there is a gap, the mattress is probably too hard: if you cannot push your hand in easily, the bed is too soft.
- Roll from side to side. If it is difficult to roll, the mattress is too soft.
- Have enough width to turn to and fro and roll over – 91.5 cm (36 in) is recommended for a single bed.

BENDING

Bending down is considered to be the primary hazard responsible for the damage which causes lower back pain. (See **backache**, **disc pro-lapse**, **pain**.)

Certain activities may require prolonged for-ward bending, stooping or **flexion** of the back for example:

- *Gardening*.
- *Vacuuming*.
- Scrubbing the kitchen floor.
- Cleaning *teeth*.
- Shaving.

Bending is controlled by the *muscles*, the *ligaments* and the facet joints of the *vertebrae* of the lower back which allow forward movement. It is therefore important to keep the back supple in order to prevent damage and allow easy bending. (See *mobilising exercises*.)

Tips when bending

- Always bend your hips and knees and keep your back straight if you are *lifting* an object.
- Bend the knees as much as possible and squat or half squat. (See *squatting*.)
- Use long-handled tools in the house and garden if you have recurrent backache from bending down. (See *gardening*.)
- Every five minutes stand upright and bend backwards five or six times to restore the lumbar curve and alter the angle of the lumbar region. (See *curves*, *extension*, *lordosis*.)
- Kneel when making the bed, vacuuming, cleaning the floor or weeding the garden. (See *bedding*, *housework*, *gardening*.)

NOTE: If you have *acute pain*, avoid bending forwards as you will be forced to lose the low back curve.

BIOMECHANICS

Biomechanics is the study of the effects of *stress* on the body during everyday activities.

The mechanics of the back have to be understood in the same way as those of a car if you want the back to operate efficiently. *Bones*, *ligaments* and *discs* react to a load being applied, up to a certain limit; when the load is removed they return to their initial shape.

However, there is a limit beyond which damage will result. Repeated small stresses have a cumulative effect not dissimilar to metal fatigue and may accelerate the ageing process of the back, which will in turn reduce the back's ability to withstand stress and strain.

It is possible to estimate the amount of stress put on the back when *lifting* or moving objects in different ways. This will vary, depending on how the objects are moved, as well as their weight and size. For example, the pressure on the structures of the back can be significantly reduced by avoiding bending and twisting movements during the lift and by careful planning and timing. The stress is also reduced by the natural supporting mechanism supplied by the tensing of the *abdominal muscles*.

BLEEDING

This may occur in the joints of the back when *inflammation* results from an accident or injury.

BLOCKING

An expression used to describe a difference in the movement between one joint and its neighbour, as felt by a manipulator. (See *manipulation*.)

BLOOD

See *circulation*.

BLOOD TESTS

A blood sample taken by the doctor or the pathology laboratory in the hospital will be necessary to diagnose certain diseases of the back, for example *ankylosing spondilitis* and *rheumatoid arthritis*. A blood count is done of the various cells which make up the blood and the erythocyte sedimentation rate of the blood (ESR) is established to show whether infection or chronic inflammation is present.

BONE

Bone is one of the hardest structures in the body but contrary to popular belief it is not solid. Bone is formed by a process called ossification and it is constantly being reformed and remoulded during life. Hard bone forms the surface layer and spongy more porous bone containing bone marrow is found inside this hard bone.

It is important to understand that bone mass increases in childhood and continues into adult life, when the process slows down and it goes into reverse in later life. In order to ensure that you have strong bones, an adequate intake of calcium, phosphorus compounds and Vitamin D is essential for the normal growth of bone.

The bones of the back, the **vertebrae**, **sacrum** and **coccyx**, vary in shape and differ considerably according to heredity, lifestyle and the various strains and stresses to which they are subjected every day. There are many disorders of bone which may affect the back. A bone may be 'out of place', an expression often used by manipulators (such as **chiropractors** or **osteopaths**), but it is difficult to prove unless it shows on an X-ray. Bones can be broken – fractured by an accident or an injury – and they can degenerate by the process of **osteo-arthrosis** and when the bones become less calcified and more porous in later life, a process called **osteoporosis**.

BOTTOM

The **muscles** of the bottom are called the gluteal muscles and their **tone** is extremely important for maintaining the upright **posture** of the trunk on the hips and legs, for the stability of the back and for the prevention of damage to the **lumbar region**. The muscles enable you to climb, and run, and they support the posture of the spine in **standing** and **walking**.

The **pelvic tilt** exercise is excellent for toning the muscles of your bottom and you can do this exercise at the bus stop, in a traffic jam, or while waiting in the queue at the checkout in the supermarket!

BOWLERS' BACK

Cricketers often suffer with back problems as often they do not have proper warm ups. Bowlers' backs suffer from **arching**, leaning backwards and the outswing action. (See **spondy-lolisthesis**, **lumbar region**.)

BRA

See **clothing**.

BRACES

Braces are used in the early stages for corrective treatment of pronounced **curves** of the lumbar and thoracic regions of the back. Severe cases of **scoliosis** may necessitate the daily wearing of a Milwaukee brace, which is only removed for corrective exercises and bathing. Braces are cumbersome appliances, but can be very effective if worn as instructed by the medical consultant.

BRACHIALGIA

If a **disc** in the **neck** region bulges sideways, pressing on a nerve root as it leaves the spinal canal, it causes pain in the arm and hand. There may be 'pins and needles' or numbness, and the arm can feel weak.

What to do

- Rest and seek medical advice.
- Wear a **collar** for support.
- Have treatment, which may consist of **manipulation** and **mobilisation** techniques or neck **traction** to relieve the pressure.

BRAIN

The brain and the **spinal cord** form the central **nervous system**. The brain is like a combination of a telephone exchange and the most complicated computer-like structure that is known to man; it relays messages, interprets them and reacts to problems using the nerves like telephone wires to send messages all over the body. It is encased in the bony skull and is comparatively heavy. It connects with the spinal cord at the top of the back, in the region of the small cervical vertebrae, so good **posture** and support are essential if nerve pathways are to remain open.

BREATHING EXERCISES

Correct breathing will promote muscular relaxation and keep the thoracic joints mobile. All back exercises should be done with regular deep breathing; inhale through the nose before beginning an exercise and then exhale through the mouth while doing the most strenuous part, concentrating all the time.

Two exercises

Lie on your back on a firm surface with the head and neck supported on a pillow and with the hips and knees bent at a comfortable angle, keeping the feet flat on the floor.

- Put your hands on your ribs at the sides of your chest. Breathe in deeply through your nose and think about the movement, so you feel your lungs filling up like a pair of balloons, so they push the ribs out against your hands. Breathe out through your mouth, squeezing your hands against the ribs to push the air out and expel all the waste products.
- Put one hand on the soft spot between the ribs at the front of the chest, where the diaphragm can be felt, and the other on top of the chest to hold it still. Breathe in

through your nose until you feel the bottom hand rising, then breathe out through your mouth, sighing gently and pushing your hand down on the soft spot. Repeat each exercise slowly five times.

NOTE: Practise deep breathing several times a day for relaxation and relief from tension.

BRONCHITIS

This chest condition – **inflammation** (*itis*) of the tubes in the **lungs** (*bronchi*) – can cause pain in the back because the breathing mechanism is involved. Muscle **spasm, pain** and rigidity can occur.

- Seek medical advice from the doctor.
- Keep warm and stay indoors.
- Do **breathing exercises**.
- Have inhalations using Friar's Balsam or Karvol.
- Get plenty of rest.

BRUISING

A bruised back can be extremely painful and may persist for some weeks. (See **acute back**, **backache**, **coccydinia**.)

BUCKET CHAIRS

See **chairs**.

BURSITIS

A bursa is a liquid-filled sac which performs a lubricating and shock absorbing function. It thus helps muscles as they slide over bone, preventing fraying and tears. Pain in the thigh radiating into the buttock and low back, or pain down the arm, may be due to *inflammation* in the bursa of a hip or shoulder joint.

BUTTOCKS

See *bottom*.

CALCIUM

This mineral is essential for the maintenance of **bone** since it is one of its chief constituents. (See also **vitamins**.)

CALF MUSCLES

The calf muscles are key **muscles** for **posture**, especially in people who stand all day wearing high heels or for those who like **jogging**. Shortened calf muscles should be gently stretched for good posture and correct **walking**.

Exercise for calf muscles

Stand comfortably with your feet about 12 in (30 cm) apart. Place one foot in front of your body and one behind, with the toes pointing forwards.

Lower the body by bending the front knee. Keep the back leg straight and both feet on the floor. You will feel a stretch in the calf muscle of the back leg. Keep your back straight while you are doing this exercise. Repeat the exercise five times for each leg, pushing gently a little further each time.

CANCER

Cancer can be one of the causes of **back pain**. The pain is usually constant and not related to movement, posture or activities. Cancer of the bone is usually noted on X-rays and later in various scans. Weight loss, tiredness and a poor appetite are other signs which accompany the constant pain, and medical direction is imperative.

CARRYING

Never carry anything if the back is aching or painful or if back pain is experienced intermittently – leave it to other people. A load of school books, a shopping bag or a heavy briefcase, carried on one side of the body, can cause leaning to that side resulting in a sideways curve or *scoliosis* which will cause **compression** and **pain**. (See **lifting, bags**).

Rules for carrying

- Think about how you are going to carry an object and concentrate while you are performing the action so you do not strain your back.
- Always divide a large weight into two smaller weights of equal size.

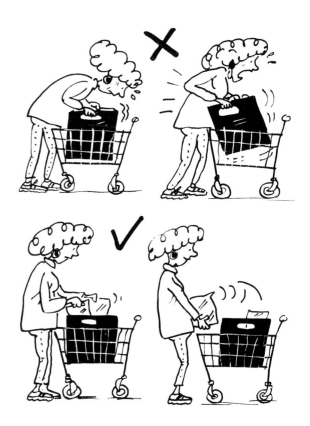

- Carry an equal amount on each side, or balance it on the shoulders.
- Carry the object close to the body in a balanced fashion, never held away from you.
- Use a trolley, hoist or **sling** if it makes carrying easier.
- Always ask supermarket or railway staff to help with shopping or luggage to avoid back twinges from heavy loads.

CARS

This form of transport has steadily become more popular, and many of us spend a proportion of every day driving a car. A supportive car seat is therefore essential as the comfort of the driver has a part to play in safety on the road; if you are seated uncomfortably, the back becomes stiff, the neck and shoulder muscles ache and you become tired and less attentive, which in turn leads to situations where accidents can happen.

Choose a car carefully, spending time to find one that suits your back as well as your budget; a smart fashionable car is no good if you are very tall and have to sit wedged under the roof or if you have to lie down in a racing driver position, suffering the vibrations of uneven roads. Car manufacturers are now much more aware that firm seating with good thigh support is essential. Test several cars when purchasing a new one in order to see which one is most comfortable for your back; remember no two individuals are the same. Power assisted steering is an important asset if you have a bad back; while an automatic transmission is advisable if you have chronic back pain. If necessary a specialised seat can be fitted to any car to give the driver a relaxed, supportive comfortable position.

Tips for travelling in the car

- On long-distance journeys, take frequent breaks – a short walk or stretch in order to relieve the strain on the back from sitting in one position for too long is essential. (See **sitting**, **walking**.)
- Bottom tightening and relaxing can prevent stiffness if performed when the car is stationary. (See **pelvic tilt**.)
- A softly sprung short car seat with an upright or sagging back will not give good support. If you make the car seat more rigid and support the lumbar curve, it will help. There are several cushions specially made to support the back in the car, such as a Backfriend by MeDesign, a Putnam's Backrest or a McKenzie Lumbar Roll. (See **chairs**, **supports**.)
- Adjust the car seat so your legs are slightly bent. The legs should never be straight with the knees locked when you are touching the control pedals as the structures in the back will become overstretched and nerve pain can result.
- Learn to get in and out of the car correctly so you avoid undue pressure on the **vertebrae** and **discs**. (See **compression**). Keep the knees together, get in backwards by sitting on the edge of the seat, using the thigh muscles to swing the legs slowly and gently round into the car. Reverse the procedure when getting out of the car. Alternatively, step in with one leg, keeping the other leg bent. Keep the knees close together and swivel on the one foot and the toes to get round into the seat.

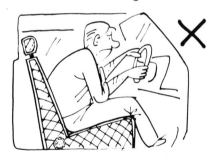

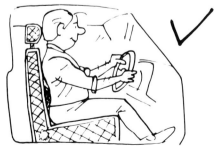

- Try and eliminate unnecessary **tension** while driving. Never drive with straight arms; relax the **shoulders** and **neck** muscles so you do not hunch and peer over the steering wheel. Lightly grip the wheel, and in stationary traffic practise raising and rotating the shoulders gently backwards. (See **posture**.)
- If you have back pain and are in the passenger seat, the arms can be supported on a **cushion** or pillow on the lap to avoid a drag on the neck, arms and upper back.
- Make sure you have clear vision through a clean windscreen so that you do not have to peer out and strain the back.
- If back pain is present, sit in the front seat to avoid maximum **vibration** and **jarring** as there is more room to stretch the legs. The seat should fully support the thighs.
- The rear seat is useful for travelling when back pain is so severe that sitting is no longer tolerable; the passenger can recline with the hips and knees flexed and supported by **pillows**, while a lumbar **corset**, such as a **Flexfit**, or a neck **collar** can be worn for extra support. **Kneeling** is also a good position in the back seat if you find sitting or lying painful.

NOTE: It is better NOT to travel if you have an **acute back**.

CARTILAGE

Cartilage is a gristle-like elastic tissue which is softer and less rigid than bone. It is found on the articular surfaces of the bones where they move over each other in the **joints**. It provides a slippery surface and acts as a shock absorber. The articulating surfaces of the facet joints of the **vertebrae** are lined with cartilage.

CAT SCAN

CAT stands for computerised axial tomography, a computer-aided scanning technique for obtain-ing an accurate examination of the body. Soft tissues show up as well as bone in the scan, making a more accurate diagnosis. If you have such a scan you will be placed on a table which moves into a tunnel equipped with the scanner, and the resulting picture will show, for example, discs and nerves as well as the vertebrae, and whether there is a disc prolapse. It is an expensive examination but is a reliable method of helping ascertain the cause of back pain.

CAUDA EQUINA

'Cauda' is Latin for tail, 'equina' for horse. The termination of the **spinal cord** as it approaches the tail bone or **coccyx** forms the cauda equina, the horse's tail.

CENTRAL NERVOUS SYSTEM

See **nervous system**.

CERVICAL MANIPULATION

See **manipulation**.

CERVICAL REGION

The cervical region or **neck** has seven **vertebrae**. They are numbered, from top to bottom, C1 to C7. The highest and smallest of these support the head.

The cervical region is very flexible due to the design of the **facet joints**, the **pivot joint** between the **atlas** and the **axis** and the complex **muscle** structure which make it possible for the head to move in a wide range.

CERVICAL SPONDYLOSIS

A general deterioration in the bones and **discs** of the neck due to the excessive use of head movements results in the condition called cervical spondylosis. (See **spondylosis**.) Movement in the neck becomes limited and this may also extend to the **shoulders** and arms. The most likely place for cervical spondylosis is in the fifth, sixth or seventh cervical **vertebrae**. It will show on an X-ray as a crumbling of the **bone**, and the **joint** spaces will be narrowed. It is most common in the 35–50 age group.

What to do

- Seek professional medical advice about treatment.
- Stop all movements that cause **pain** and rest the **neck**.
- Wear a neck **collar** to support the head.

CERVICAL TRACTION

See **traction**.

CHAIRS

'Thus first necessity invented stools,
Convenience next suggested elbow-chairs
And luxury the accomplish'd Sofa last'
William Cowper, 1731-1800

Many people spend their domestic and working lives seated, with long hours often spent in front of a VDU or television set. **Ergonomics** have made great advances in the seating posture and furniture design, but designers still have a long way to go and most of the chairs you use every day are designed with little thought for the shape of the body and the need to support the back.

Your back is not straight but S curved, and a straight upright chair causes you to lose this curve, increasing the pressure on the **discs** and bones in the lower back. If you try to move forwards on this chair to work at a desk or table, the back will assume a C curve. However, there are many types of chair on the market now, designed to achieve the correct sitting **posture**.

Selecting a chair

There is no single chair that is right for everybody, although many are very adaptable. The correct selection will depend on the following:

- The height and shape of your back; that is, the degree of curve in your **cervical**, **thoracic** and **lumbar region**.
- The depth of the seat, which should provide adequate thigh support but not give any pressure on the back of the thighs. A padded sloping front edge to the chair is beneficial for preventing the constriction of blood vessels under the thighs. (See **compression**, **crossed legs**.)
- The backrest of the chair should allow mobility of the lumbar and pelvic regions so that you maintain a good **circulation** if it is necessary to sit for long periods.
- An adjustable lumbar support for the chair and a forward tilting seat angle of 8–10 degrees for bending forwards to work at a desk are ergonomically essential, so that your eyes are in line with your work. (See **housework**, **office**, **visual display unit**, **work**.)
- The chair should be comfortable and firm allowing you to have a good sitting posture and your feet to touch the floor. Use a footstool if necessary.
- Have a chair with armrests, as they can assist you with getting in and out of the chair.

NOTE: It is essential to take time when choosing a chair. Your comfort depends on the final decision.

How to get into a chair

- Place one or two firm cushions on the seat

of the chair if you have a bad back so you do not have too far to sit down.

- Keep your feet shoulder-width apart, so that you have a firm base and, placing one foot back under the chair, bend your knees, keeping the back straight, the tummy muscles firm and the chin tucked in.
- Turn slightly to reach for one arm of the chair.
- Place both hands on the arms of the chair, bend your knees, lower yourself slowly and sit down. Don't flop in the chair, as you will jar your back and damage the chair. (See **jarring**.)

Getting out of a chair

- Place your feet at the edge of the chair or if possible slightly underneath.
- Move forwards to the edge of the chair.
- Tighten your abdominal and bottom muscles (see **pelvic tilt**) and, pushing on your arms, straighten your **knees**, tightening the thigh muscles, and stand up slowly.
- If you are not confident about standing up without looking at the floor, either look down with your nose over your toes, or have a sturdy table near the armchair to help you get up.

BACKFRIEND

The MeDesign Backfriend is the brainchild of a British physician, Dr Duncan Troup, who is an international authority on back problems. It consists of a moulded back rest and seat, foam padded for extra comfort, and weighs less than 4 lb (1.8 kg.) The frame is rigid and therefore does not sag or roll, maintaining a firm position whenever you use it. It can be used on any seat or chair so a comfortable position for the back is possible when travelling, at the cinema, visiting friends or at work, thereby avoiding the need for numerous cushions. (See **air travel**, **cars**, **office**, **supports**, **workplace**.) It folds flat and has a built-in carrying grip. For extra comfort and warmth, a sheepskin cover is available.

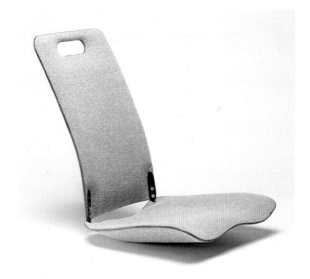

The MeDesign Backfriend

Chairs for the home

Armchairs
There is a wide range of choice for this very relaxing fireside chair. A good seat height and correctly shaped back with a firm lumbar support and a contoured front edge, preventing pressure under the thighs, are all essential. The back rest should be high enough to support the **shoulders** and **neck** region but it should allow for normal head movements. Make sure the chair is wide enough for activities such as knitting and reading, and if you have backache do not choose a sagging armchair. A space under an armchair is helpful for positioning the feet when getting in and out.

There are now armchairs for the elderly and disabled that have a mechanical tilting seat to help you stand, but these should not be used unless the supportive muscles of the back are very weak and unable to lift the body weight.

Bucket chairs
These saggy chairs will aggravate a bad back since there is very little support and the hammock effect will cause strain when getting in and out of the chair.

do not use the traditional vertical and horizontal design, but allow the pelvis to tip forwards so very little weight goes through the lower back. The back assumes the S curves of good **posture** automatically but strain can be felt on the knees and shins, especially if **arthritis** is present. (See **Balans, Mandal**.)

Reclining chairs
If you enjoy reclining, invest in a chair that fully supports your legs and keeps your knees higher than your hips, with a shaped lumbar support. Your shoulders should not be pushed forwards and the neck must be adequately supported.

The **BALANS** TRIPOS from Stokke is an all-purpose reclining chair, since it has three positions to choose from depending on your mood. In the first position you have an 'alternative seating' chair; tilt it back once and you have a comfortable position for reading; for relaxation tilt it right back and you are fully supported.

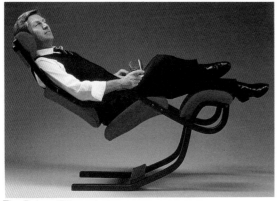

The Balans Tripos chair

Rocking chairs
These chairs provide mobility for the back and therefore help maintain a good circulation. As the late President John F. Kennedy discovered following a back injury, these are good chairs if you have a back problem as the rocking motion is pleasant, relaxing and keeps you mobile.

The **BALANS** PENDULUM is a chair developed by Stokke that follows your movements, whether leaning forwards or rocking backwards. The back stretcher serves as arms for the chair and the back rest gives support

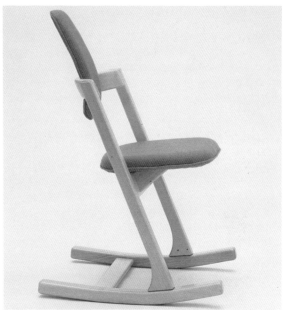

The Balans Pendulum chair

between the shoulder blades, freeing the chest and enabling you to breathe easily. The freedom of this rocking chair makes it versatile for both use at home in a dining room or working in the office.

Sofas
Deep low sofas are usually squashy, uncomfortable and have somewhat bulky cushions. They put the back into a C curve and are impossible to get out of when you want to stand up. Avoid all low soft sofas whenever possible.

Straight-back chairs
These vertical upright chairs with a horizontal seat make you sit upright, but put a strain on the back and encourage a round back and shoulders. A lumbar **support** will make this type of chair more comfortable. On a horizontal seat, use a footstool to allow the knees to be slightly higher than the hips. (See **Putnam, support, wedge**.)

Traditional chairs with sloping backs
These chairs are more comfortable since the seat usually slopes towards the rear of the chair. This enables you to use the backrest for lumbar support.

Office chairs

These should have a good simple design with easy-to-work controls. The backrest should encourage good **posture** and preferably there should be a space between the seat and the bottom of the backrest, unless a sacral support is necessary.

LABOMATIC WORKING CHAIR

A range of chairs specially developed by two experts, designer Jacob Jensen and the ergonomist Vibeke Leschly, from Denmark. Its seat is wide, deep and well contoured. The back rest is also large, which helps give extra support and comfort. It has automatic height adjustment and the seat can be set at any angle from −4 to +10 degrees. The Labomatic seat actually moves due to a weight-activated hydraulic cylinder that controls the movement of the seat. As soon as you sit on the chair, your body weight forces the cylinder to compress, which causes the angle of the seat to change automatically and constantly. As a result the muscles in the back remain active, avoiding stiffness. The chair has curved adjustable arm rests. Its computerised mechanism can quickly adapt to any build, making it ideal for anyone working at a desk.

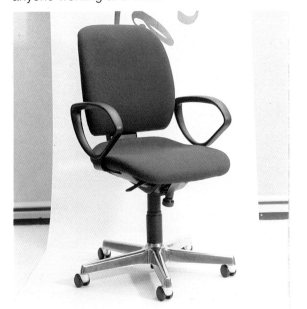

Labomatic working chair

CREDO CHAIR

This chair, designed by Peter Opsvik and developed by Hag in Norway, has a free-floating seat to allow you to tilt forwards and backwards, without any adjustment, to secure a natural sitting posture. The chair adapts to you, not vice versa. The useful slide action of the seat makes the chair suitable for people of varying heights and leg lengths.

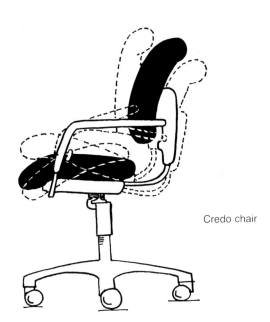

Credo chair

ERGOFORM WORKSEAT

This innovative chair has been developed in Canada by a team including a professor of industrial design and a chiropractor. It is hinged at the base of the seat, and supports the back in every position on a forward-inclining seat surface, which is important for maintaining the natural lumbar curve while working at a desk. The back remains in full contact with the central column of the chair at all times. It allows for complete manoeuvrability at the workplace because the base rotates a full 360 degrees without manual adjustment, giving you full access to everything within reach. It can be adjusted to accommodate children or adults.

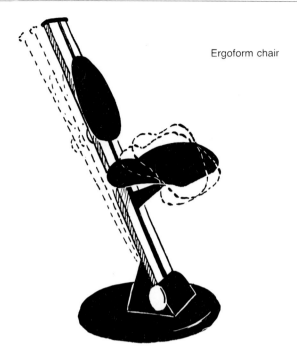

Ergoform chair

SPINE SEAT

This kneeling chair is the branchild of Harry Hepburn and Hugh Slater, (principal of the West London School of Reflexology), who felt that the current range of kneeling chairs did not provide

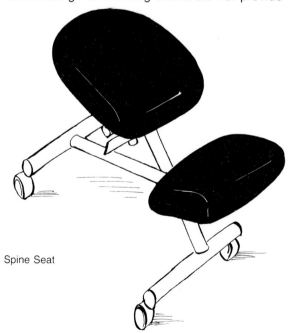

Spine Seat

enough adjustability. The Spine Seat provides length adjustment to cater for people with varying leg lengths, a manual height adjustment to suit various work heights and a wide, comfortable seat that has an independent tilt mechanism.

CHARTERED PHYSIOTHERAPIST

See **physiotherapy**

CHILDBIRTH

During childbirth the mother may experience severe **backache** and even **pain**, due to the strong expulsive contractions of the uterus causing **compression** on the structures of the back.

It is very important to find a delivery position which is practised well in advance so that it is as comfortable and as natural as possible. Such a position will prevent an excessive load on tense back muscles and avoid strain on weak overstretched **abdominal muscles**. The neck should be well supported with **pillows** or a cervical roll, especially during the second stage of labour. Typical positions are:

- Side lying.
- Half squatting.
- Lying with the legs elevated and supported in slings, with the hips and knees at 90 degrees flexion.

Backache can be eased in the early stages of childbirth by **massage** or by stroking the lower back with the heel of the hand. This can either be done by yourself or by enlisting the help of a sympathetic partner. During childbirth itself anaesthesia of the lower part of the body, including the back, is possible with an **epidural injection**.

It is advisable to attend antenatal classes, where childbirth topics are discussed fully and where various positions can be learnt in preparation for childbirth. The address of the National Childbirth Trust, the Royal College of Midwives and the Association of Chartered Physiotherapists in Obstetrics and Gynaecology can be found in the Where To Get Help section at the end of the book.

CHIROPODY

This is the study and care of the feet, including the structure and disorders. Treatment is carried out by a trained practitioner called a chiropodist. (See **podiatrist**.)

CHIROPRACTIC

Chiropractic means 'practice with the hands', being derived from the Greek words *cheir*, hand, and *praktikos*, done by. Chiropractic is manipulative treatment for misalignments of the back and its joints which can lead to other complaints. (See **manipulation**.) It was developed in the late 1800s by Daniel Palmer of Davenport, Iowa, a grocer turned 'magnetic healer'.

Modern chiropractic is the branch of **complementary medicine** which specialises in the mechanical disorders of the **joints**, particularly the spinal joints, and their effects on the **nervous system**.

The difference between chiropractic and **osteopathy** is that an osteopath mostly treats the affected back joints, searching for a lack of mobility by levering and twisting manipulations, whereas a chiropractor is more exact, feeling for individual vertebral displacements with specific thrusting techniques at one level, applied directly to the misaligned bone after a diagnostic X-ray.

Chiropractor

A qualified chiropractor receives training which varies from four to seven years according to the legal requirements of the country where he or she has trained. The object of treatment is for the chiropractor to improve the mobility of the spine and relax the surrounding muscles. This profession is recognised by the letters DC, doctor of chiropractic.

In the UK it is advisable to choose a registered member of the British Chiropractors Association (see Where To Get Help section at the end of the book).

CHRISTMAS

In order to have a happy Christmas:

- Avoid **carrying** lots of heavy Christmas shopping and parcels. Take care when getting parcels in and out of car.
- When putting up decorations and stretching the **neck** to hang the lights on a high Christmas tree, have a stable extending ladder or two chairs. (See **decorating**.)
- Carry the turkey carefully. It may weigh over 20 lb, so ask a man in the family to lift it in and out of the oven and remind him to observe the rules for **lifting**.
- Don't slump in front of the television after a heavy lunch; go for a good walk. This will avoid a stiff neck and indigestion! (See **chairs, walking**.)

CHRONIC BACK

A **backache** or **pain** that persists for a long time is said to be chronic. Chronic back problems occur either:

- as a result of the direct continuation of **acute back** pain in which the irritant has grown milder; or
- as the result of a minor irritant which is not enough to cause an acute reaction.

Chronic backache may never completely disappear. It is a state that shows no change or a very slow change over a period of time. However, the severity, duration and region of the pain may vary due to the fibrous tissue which forms, with subsequent loss of elasticity and mobility, leading to **stress** and muscle **spasm**.

Some causes of chronic back pain are:

- Muscular spasm and tension.
- Poor **posture**.

- *Disc prolapse*.
- Joint and ligament **strain**.
- **Ligament** injuries.
- **Scoliosis**.
- Old age.

What to do

Consult a specialist; this may be an orthopaedic surgeon or neurosurgeon, a neurologist or rheumatology specialist. They will conduct various tests, such as blood tests, X-rays and scans, and you may be referred for treatment to a chartered **physiotherapist**, an **osteopath** or a **chiropractor**. Drugs, injections and surgery may be necessary. However, by following the instructions for acute back problems, and trying to find the cause of the chronic back pain, you may be able to help yourself.

- Stop **lifting** and **carrying** except for very light objects.
- Use a trolley, hoist or **sling** where it will help.
- Wear a **corset** or **collar** until you can strengthen your muscles by **exercise**.
- Check your **bed**, **chairs** and **car** seat; they may need replacing.
- Walk for at least ten minutes every day. (See **walking**.)
- Learn to relax. (See **relaxation**.)
- Learn simple **massage** techniques.

See the Where To Get Help and Suggested Further Reading sections at the back of the book.

NOTE: You should not expect a chronic back to get better quickly; judge your healing time by the length of time you've had the symptoms.

CIRCULATION

The movement of blood from the heart round the body and back to the heart again takes place in arteries and veins. In the back the blood vessels travel in spinal pathways, up and down the vertebrae. If there should be bony encroachment or displacement of a disc in the back, it may cause pressure on the vessels, resulting in circulatory problems.

Arterial flow

Blood flowing out from the heart circulates through the arteries, with the pumping pressure of the heart behind it to propel it forwards.

Veinous flow

There is no pumping pressure for the return flow through the veins to the heart. The circulation of the venous blood relies on the contractions of the large muscles of the arms, lower back and legs to pump the blood in a rhythmic continuous fashion back to the heart. Valves in the veins prevent the blood flowing the wrong way.

Exercise and the circulation

Muscular activity, which relies on the oxygen carried in the bloodstream for its energy, is thus vitally important and is unfortunately minimised with modern sedentary living. Fatigue, the sensation of dragging on the legs, weariness in the back, cramp and, in extreme cases, fainting, are due to inadequate circulation, resulting in lack of oxygen and leaving waste products stagnating in the tissues.

What to do

- Don't sit for too long at a **desk**, a **VDU** or in front of the **television**.
- Get up, stretch and move your legs frequently.
- Never sit with **crossed legs**.
- Don't drive if you can walk or cycle. **Exercise** and activities such as **walking, swimming** and **cycling** are all good for the circulation, but in moderation according to your age.

For maintaining a good circulation by regular exercise this table will help.

Age	Time	Exercise	Duration
20–30	3 days a week	Intensive work out	1 hour
30–40	3 days a week	Less intensive	1 hour
40–50	Alternate days	At a reasonable pace	1 hour
50–60	6 days a week	Regular pace	½ – ¾ hour
Over 60	Every day	Gently	For as long as you like

Increase the frequency and decrease the intensity of exercise to maintain a healthy circulation.

CLASSES

See **back school**.

CLOTHING

It is not necessary to be fashionable at the expense of your back. You should dress comfortably and avoid restrictive clothing. And if you have problems with dressing, several products are available which may help you – for example, a 'helping hand' grabber or a long-handled shoehorn.

Bras

Women with heavy breasts can suffer from severe upper back and shoulder pain if they do not wear a correctly sized well-designed bra. The pain may radiate into the **neck** and **shoulders**, causing rigidity in the **thoracic region** and poor **posture** – perhaps due to an ill-fitting shallow bra with narrow straps that dig into the skin and muscles.

It is essential to have a well-fitted bra with straps at least an inch (2·5 cm) wide if problems are to be prevented. Take time, and use the help of a shop assistant, to try on a range of bras so you are comfortable – it will be worth any extra expense.

If you have back pain:

- either put on a bra back to front, fastening the hooks while they are in front; or
- put the straps over the shoulders, leaning forwards with one foot raised on a low stool, and fasten it in this position.

Corsets and girdles

Corsets and **girdles** can be worn to support the back, but if they are only worn for vanity and to make the tummy flatter, this will result in weak and wasted muscles.

Trousers and skirts

Avoid wearing tight restrictive trousers or tights if your back is painful; it will be difficult to get them on and off.

Wear a skirt that does not cause you embarrassment; for example, a miniskirt that makes you walk with bent knees and a curved back is obviously not a good idea. (See **curves**.)

Nightclothes

Nightclothes should not constrict movement and should be warm, in case bedclothes fall off during the night allowing a draught on the back. (See **bedding**.)

COCCYDINIA

The **coccyx** rarely gives problems, except perhaps after a heavy fall such as:

- When a chair is pulled away from under you.
- You have a heavy fall downstairs.
- A horse riding accident.
- A skiing injury.

Any such damage is called coccydinia and can be extremely painful; bruising can last for several months, preventing you from sitting comfortably. If severe pain continues, an injection may be given to reduce **inflammation**, but if there is a **fracture**, then surgery may be necessary. Such surgery involves removing any severed fragments, but it is fairly minor and you will be walking again when the wound has healed. When sitting, a circular rubber or foam ring with a hole for the tail will relieve pressure on the *coccyx*.

COCCYX

The four small bones that are fused together at the base of the back is the tail or coccyx. (See *anatomy*.)

COD LIVER OIL

Cod liver oil provides *vitamins* that are essential for building strong *bones* in growing children.

COLDS

Colds can cause back pain. Muscular spasm can occur very suddenly in the lower back if you have been sitting in a cold *draught* causing temporary *acute pain*. (See *coughing, sneezing*.)

COLD THERAPY

While most people prefer and get relief by treating back pain with heat, some get quicker relief with cold applications, for example in the form of crushed ice, cold wet towels, an ethyl chloride spray, or a cold gel pack. (See *acute back*.)

Heat is more comfortable as it expands the blood vessels. Cold does just the opposite; the blood vessels at first become constricted. However after a period of time, usually five to ten minutes, the constricted vessels become tired, relax and dilate.

Cold can be a shock initially. A burning tingling sensation will be felt during the cooling process, but after the first few minutes of being uncomfortable the area to which the cold is applied becomes numb and it is then accompanied by a marvellous sensation of relief from *pain*.

What to do

- Oil the area of skin, to avoid any chance of an ice burn.
- Wrap the ice in a towel before applying it to the painful area.
- Watch the skin carefully for any sign of irritation.
- Apply it for a maximum of 10 to 15 minutes, three times a day.
- The cold pack should cover an area larger than the site of the pain.
- Try gentle *mobilising exercises* once the cold application is removed.
- Take care if you use a cold spray – they are inflammable!

NOTE: Never apply ice directly to the skin. Anyone with a heart problem should not apply cold therapy.

COLD WRAP

A flexible Cold Wrap from *Spenco* is a convenient way of treating acute back conditions with cold therapy. It contains hydroflex gel, and is stored in the freezer for instant use. The gel ensures it remains flexible and doesn't ice up, and it gives an even distribution of cold.

COLITIS

It sometimes happens that the only pain produced by colitis, inflammation of the colon or large intestine, is back pain. Pain radiates from the colon along the nerve pathways and produces pain in the back. (See *backache, referred pain*.) If this occurs, seek a medical opinion immediately.

COLLARS

Collars are a valuable support, for an acute *neck* or an upper back problem, since the head is heavy and the neck without total support cannot cope, for example in such conditions as:

- A *whiplash* injury.
- A wry neck or torticollis.
- Severe arm problems.
- *Headaches*.
- A *fracture*.

Collars are not the most glamorous of appliances being made of felt, foam, plaztazote, plastic or plaster of Paris.

- Collars should be fitted correctly by a medical practitioner so that they offer good firm support. Learn how to wear a collar by asking for instructions.
- It is advisable to start gentle movements within 48 hours to prevent stiffness and further spasm. (See *exercise*, *neck*.)
- A collar should not be worn for too long as the *muscles* will waste if they are not exercised regularly.
- A scarf tied like a man's stock or cravat can help conceal a collar, which may have to be worn for anything from 48 hours to three months, according to the problem.
- Coloured stockings can also be pulled over the collar to match clothes.

COMMUNICATION

Good communication is vital if back *pain* is to be prevented. Ignorance and hoping the pain will go away will not produce results and is extremely negative. The media, advertising and many publications describe and discuss back problems; however it is important to talk to your doctor and any other medical practitioner – ask questions and expect answers in order to establish the causes of your problems and how to prevent them in the future. See Suggested Further Reading.

COMPLEMENTARY MEDICINE

Complementary or alternative medicine covers many different therapies. They can be used in place of (as alternatives to) or alongside (complementary to) conventional medicine. *Alexander Technique*, *osteopathy*, *chiropractic* and *reflexology* are some of the complementary therapies.

The difference between conventional orthodox medicine and complementary medicine is that while conventional medicine emphasises treating the particular disease of a person, based on scientific facts, complementary medicine emphasises treating a person's health and general well-being as a whole and is known as a holistic approach. Conventional medical practitioners now frequently adopt complementary medical techniques. (See the Where To Get Help section for the addresses of the appropriate organisations.)

COMPRESSION

Nerve root compression, due to a *disc* protrusion or a disc prolapse, causes pain and there will be subsequent muscle spasm in the back which can travel to the arms and legs. If a nerve is compressed for an extended period it eventually stops causing pain as the nerve swells, and numbness will result.

The two most common conditions which occur as a result of compression are:

- *Sciatica* in the leg caused by compression of the sciatic nerve.
- *Brachialgia* in the arm caused by compression of the brachial nerve.

CONGENITAL DEFECTS

Abnormalities of the back do sometimes take place at or before birth; for example, the *spinal canal* can be narrower than it ought to be, and it can also vary in shape so the nerves become compressed at an early age. (See *compression*.) Often the back pain is associated with such a congenital abnormality, but is not due to the abnormality itself. (See *abnormal back*.) The pain is usually from the unusual stresses imposed by the abnormality on the surrounding structures, especially the muscles. *Corsets*, *braces* and muscle strengthening *exercises*, under the instruction of a medical practitioner, can be beneficial, without recourse to surgery.

CONSTIPATION

See **acute back**, **toilets**.

CONSULTANT

Any medical practitioner can be consulted for information and advice about back problems. It is usual for the patient to visit the consultant unless it is an emergency. However, the consultants' medical qualifications, registration and relevant experience in back treatment should be established before a visit.

COPPER BRACELETS

Many people seem to obtain benefit by wearing a copper bracelet. Documentation and scientific evidence are sparse, but a chemical reaction appears to be induced through the skin by the copper which sometimes seems to have a beneficial effect for the relief of back symptoms.

COPY HOLDER

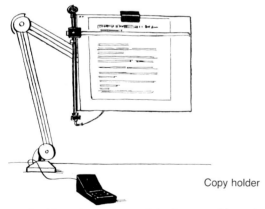

Copy holder

This product is extremely useful when working at a horizontal **desk** surface, in front of a typewriter or **visual display unit**. (See **workplace**.) It holds the copy – the sheets of paper you are working from – in a position so that you have a comfortable angle of vision and avoid **strain** on the **neck** and **lumbar region** from too much bending forwards. A copy holder is essential for typists, barristers, editors and authors, and all other occupations where a great deal of paperwork is involved at a desk or table. (See **office, writing slope**.)

CORSETS

Corsets are essential if you have a bad back. They provide an instant support for the muscles of the **lower back**, which may be in spasm, and assist the weak **abdominal muscles**.

Traditionally, corsets were made from steel bands and fabric, but methods of construction have changed over the years, and there is now a varied selection on the market. A corset should be chosen carefully and fit well. (See **Flexfit**.)

What the corset will do

- It is an instant support but a short-term solution.
- It helps intra-abdominal pressure and weak **abdominal muscles**.
- It retains a certain amount of heat, providing warmth for the back.
- It gives confidence whilst you are in pain.
- It will help a chronic back problem by giving support against **vibration** and **jarring** when travelling and during daily activities.

NOTE: You should never rely solely on corset support, but continue regular exercise to strengthen your muscles.

COST

Back pain costs the government, industry and individuals, millions of pounds every year; for example, one surgical operation costs thousands of pounds, and subsequent treatments, drugs and injections cost just as much.

Maintenance costs for a bad back

If you have regular attacks of backache or pain, take a moment to assess the cost of putting the problem right.

£

- Income lost due to days off work.
- Holiday that you have paid for and can't take.
- Private insurance costs for medical treatment.
- Treatment costs if no insurance.
- Cost of supports and equipment.
- Cost of a new bed.
- Cost of a new chair.
- Taxes for National Health Service.
- Chauffeur's or taxi costs if unable to drive.
- Cost of drugs.
- Cost of a surgical operation.
- Cost of this book.

_____

Total £

How much is it? Surely you'd enjoy spending the money elsewhere, free from back troubles?

COUGHING

A severe coughing bout, throwing the body suddenly forwards into an extreme flexed position, can cause back pain. By using the tummy muscles to stabilise the forward movement, most of the severe discomfort can be prevented. A period of relaxation should follow a coughing bout, to avoid further muscle spasm. (See **abdominal muscles**.)

COUNSELLING

Back problems, besides having physical and mechanical causes, may be due to human emotions, sexual and psychological problems. Advice is now widely available for people who wish to help themselves avoid back pain.

CRACKING

An expression used for the sudden sharp crunching noises in the bones or **joints**. **Manipula-**

tion may cause a cracking noise in the facet joints of the **vertebrae** due to the breaking down of fibrous tissue resulting from chronic **inflammation**.

CRICKING

A crick in the **neck** is another expression used to describe muscular tension in the neck leading to stiffness in the joints, discomfort and perhaps pins and needles in the arms and hands.

CROSSED LEGS

This is a bad habit – it is not good for the back or the **circulation**, and causes pressure on the nerves on the side to which you have crossed your leg. The pelvis level is tipped and the back is pulled off balance to one side, leading to **compression** of the **discs** and **joints**. Try to maintain a good balanced **posture** in sitting; if you must cross your legs, only cross them at the ankles.

CURVES

The back has a double S curve, formed at the beginning of life. The degree of the curves of the back during adult life all hinge on the **pelvic tilt** and the angle of the **sacrum**.

When there are excessive curves in the back, certain **muscles** become stretched beyond their working length and other muscles have to take up the load. This leads to acute **strain** and then chronic **backache**. (See **acute back**, **biomechanics**, **chronic back**.)

- The **lumbar** curve is called the lordotic curve. (See **lordosis**.)
- The **cervical** curve is also called a lordotic curve.
- The **thoracic** curve is called the kyphotic curve. (See **kyphosis**.)
- A lateral curve, which is called a **scoliosis**, is an abnormal sideways curve.

Use a mirror and look at your **posture** from all angles to note the degree of your individual curves.

CUSHIONS

Cushions are for comfort. They are extremely useful to provide good positioning in order to give the back plenty of support on a poor **chair** or **bed**. (See **pillows**, **positions**.)

CYCLING

Cycling is a good way to build up general fitness and maintain a healthy back. It involves the continuous and regular use of the large thigh muscles which encourages better **circulation** and results in improved heart and lung function. However, the design of the bicycle could itself be responsible for many aches and pains felt in the back, so when cycling:

- Have a suitable saddle at the right height and in the correct position for your back.

- Have a padded flexible saddle if you want to avoid **jarring**, **vibration** and subsequent pain in the bottom and pelvic region.

- Maintain an upright **posture**, using the back and **abdominal muscles** for control rather than **bending** forwards on drop handlebars in a racing position when, by over-reaching, you can stretch and strain the back.

- Distribute the weight evenly on the saddle and avoid tensing the **neck**.

- Start slowly and build up gently by taking short rides two or three times a week. (See **circulation**, **exercise**.)

- If the handlebars are too low or the frame is too small, you will get **compression** in the lower ribs.

Cycling is something all the family can enjoy and it will boost your stamina as it is a form of **aerobic** exercise. This applies also to the use of a static bicycle in the home. (See **gym**, **Tunturi**.)

DANCING

'As those move easiest who have learned to dance.'

Alexander Pope, 1688-1744

This activity can be good for the back, while ballroom dancing positively encourages good **posture**. However, **aerobic** dancing, rock and roll, the twist and one or two other modern styles of dance can be somewhat violent – frantic quick jerky movements can be too demanding on the back. Stretching and strengthening movements are good, but avoid straining and trying to overdo it in the early stages. Enjoy dancing, it will make you feel better and fitter; although when you enrol in a class check that the movements will suit your back, otherwise you may end up on a practitioner's couch! (See **ballet dancing**.)

DECOMPRESSION

This is when pressure on the nerves and blood vessels is relieved by surgery or **manipulation**. (See **compression, disc**.)

DECORATING

Painting and decorating, together with all forms of household DIY, are hazardous activities for the back and should be undertaken with careful planning to avoid **neck** and **back** pain or **strain**.

- Warm up with stretching movements before you start decorating.
- If you can, lie on planks in the style of Michelangelo painting the ceiling of the Sistine chapel, rather than stretching with the head held back to paint ceilings.

- Kneel or squat for low jobs such as painting skirting boards or plumbing under sinks. (See **knees**, **squatting**.)
- Place one foot on a stool or upturned crate when doing carpentry at a workbench.
- Make sure heights are correct for you. (See **ergonomics**.)

DEFORMITY

Structural defects resulting in back curvatures as a result of disease or at birth will cause back problems. (See **congenital defects**, **curves**). It is advisable and wise to seek immediate medical help to try and correct deformities at an early stage. The most common deformities are **scoliosis**, **lordosis**, **kyphosis** and **spondylolisthesis**.

DEGENERATION

The back degenerates with age, depending on the stresses and **strains** it has had in childhood and during your working life – and this includes housework. Degenerative changes will occur in **bone** and **discs** a great deal sooner for those continually engaged in heavy manual work, e.g. builders, farmers and nurses, or those whose back has suffered many shocks or falls due to sport or excessive activities, e.g. gymnastics, skiing, riding, motor and powerboat racing. (See **osteoarthrosis**, **osteoporosis**.)

DEHYDRATION

Loss of water content, for example in the **discs** or tissues.

DENTIST

When you visit your dentist, make sure before he starts treatment that your **neck** region is adequately supported with a small *pillow* or McKenzie Cervical Roll – if necessary take one with you. Most dentists now have special reclining chairs, but they are not designed for your individual back, so ask for a rolled up towel or cushion if there are any gaps in the neck region while you are having treatment. (See *supports*.)

DEPRESSION

Depression, *anxiety* and worry can produce a vicious circle which heightens pain and delays recovery. Although depression may not be the cause of the back *pain*, this mental state can lead to a droopy slumped *posture* resulting in lethargy and physical inactivity.

It is often hard to combat feeling low and fed up, and a doctor prescribing *anti-depressant* drugs is not always the answer. It is far more important to find the cause of the back pain and why you are depressed. (See *anger, back-ache, emotions, stress*.)

What to do

- Obtain good support from family and friends and the help of a counsellor.
- Learn *relaxation* and *breathing* exercises.
- Have regular *massage*.
- An activity such as *swimming* or *walking* may help you.
- Get a good night's sleep so *tiredness* does not lead to depression the next day.

DESKS

It is very important that desks are the right height for you when you are sitting down. At work, in the office or the schoolroom, the desk and the *chair* should allow a good working *posture*.

A desk with a sloping surface eliminates *neck* and *shoulder* strain. (See *writing slope*.) Never buy a standard fixed-height desk if you can buy an adjustable one. (See *ergonomics, workplace*.)

DIAGNOSIS

It is very important to have a diagnosis of your back problems from a qualified registered medical practitioner. This may be from a doctor, a physical medicine consultant or a surgeon; in the United Kingdom these professions are currently the only legally recognised people who are properly trained and qualified to infer from your signs and symptoms what is wrong with your back.

To give an accurate diagnosis will require a thorough examination of the back, and an *X-ray*, *blood tests*, *electromyography* or *CAT scan* may sometimes be necessary. Find out from your family doctor or the relevant professional organisation how to find an expert, and see also the Where To Get Help section at the end of the book.

DIATHERMY

Deep heat treatment may be used by a medical practitioner for the treatment of back problems. The most common form of deep heat is short-wave diathermy, in which high-frequency electro-magnetic waves produce heat in the body tissues and induce a general feeling of warmth. There are now pulsed diathermy machines, and research is showing that treatment with these machines produces beneficial results over a long period. Two or three treatments should produce a feeling of decreased stiffness and muscle relaxation. (See *electrotherapy*.)

DIET

You are what you eat, so find out what suits you. A diet consists of a balance of different nutrients and there are many books written on the subject, so make sure you have no deficiencies in your diet. (See the Suggested Further Reading list at the end of the book.)

DISC

The back is not rigid but flexible, due to shock absorbing structures between each **vertebra** and the next called intervertebral discs. They can be seen when viewing the spine from the front. These discs are engineered to deal with **compression**, preventing the vertebrae crashing, grating, grinding and rubbing against each other.

The nucleus pulposus

The core of the disc is composed of a soft jelly-like material called the nucleus pulposus. It has a shock absorber effect, working like hydraulic fluid to protect the vertebrae.

Fluid is absorbed into the disc from the surrounding tissues whilst you are asleep and squeezed out during the day when the discs are constantly under pressure from the forces of gravity when standing up, sitting, bending and lifting. During movement, however, the disc can suck in more fluid and nutrients, so if the back is sedentary and static the disc will dry out and problems will occur. (See **dehydration**, **disc prolapse**.)

Age degenerates the structure of the disc and the nucleus deteriorates from a sticky jelly-like substance to a more stringy thick consistency and it becomes more solid. (See **spondylosis**.)

The annulus

The nucleus of the disc merges strongly with the hard tough outer part of the disc, called the annulus, which encircles the central portion. The annulus has many layers in a laminated construction, formed of fibres criss-crossed at an angle, one layer lying in a slanting direction and the next layer lying in an opposite oblique direction. The annulus provides strong reinforcement to keep the vertebrae together. It minimises compression on the disc and can stretch to a limited degree, allowing flexibility in the back. If the annulus becomes twisted, the fibres are stretched and cannot cope with movement; they tear, first on

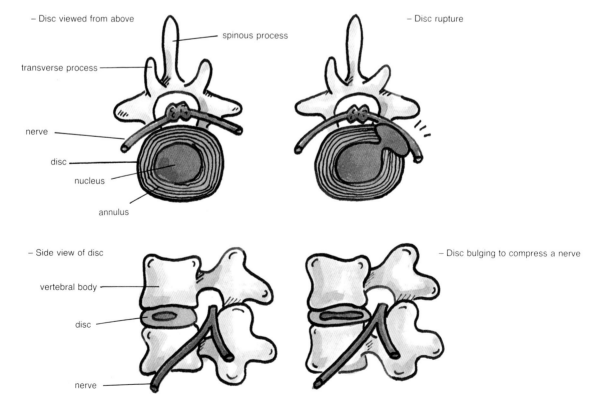

– Disc viewed from above

spinous process

transverse process

nerve

disc

nucleus

annulus

– Disc rupture

– Side view of disc

vertebral body

disc

nerve

– Disc bulging to compress a nerve

the outside layers and then on the inside, which will cause muscle *spasm* and pain in the back. (See *disc prolapse*, *pain*.)

Disc prolapse

Contrary to popular belief, a disc does NOT slip (see *slipped disc*). It becomes prolapsed due to a violent twisting action, an injury or degeneration with age. The annulus becomes so badly cracked, damaged and distorted that some of the centre or nucleus of the intervertebral disc is squeezed through the outer wall. This rupture of the annulus allows the bulging protrusion of the nucleus into the spinal canal, causing interference and pressure on the spinal cord or nerve roots. (See *compression*, *dura*.) This herniation results in severe *spasm* in the back muscles nearby and *pain* due to the compression on the sensitive spinal nerves or ligaments; there are no nerve endings in the discs themselves to cause pain. (See *referred pain*.) A prolapsed disc is most likely to occur between 25 to 50 years of age.

Disc bulge

With ageing or after injury, the contents of the disc may bulge, herniate or protrude and press on the spinal nerves. This may not necessarily cause pain. (See *compression*, *pain*.)

Disc degeneration

See *degeneration*.

Discectomy

A surgical operation on a disc.

Discogram

This technique is used to investigate a disc. After the injection of an X-ray opaque dye, *X-ray* pictures are taken to show what is happening in a disc, in order to detect a suspected disc prolapse or *degeneration*. (See *CAT scan*.)

DOCTOR

If you are a back *pain* sufferer, it is crucial to choose the right doctor. The general family practitioner has not always sufficient experience of back problems to make an accurate *diagnosis*, or there may not be time in a busy surgery for a thorough *examination*. It is therefore essential to choose a doctor who can give you advice but not a load of pills – the latter will probably relieve the pain but will not help the back problem.

However, start with your GP as he or she will have access to further investigatory tests such as an *X-ray* or *blood tests*. The doctor can then refer or recommend you to someone, such as an *orthopaedic* specialist, a *neurologist*, a chartered *physiotherapist*, a registered *osteopath* or *chiropractor*, who will help you.

Always keep your doctor informed about what you are doing for your back if you want his sympathetic ear! (See questions the *doctor* may ask.)

DRAUGHTS

Stay out of cold draughts caused by an open window or *air conditioning* since they may cool the superficial muscles of the back and cause painful *spasm*. (See *acute back*.)

DRAWING

Frequently a drawing of the back and the rest of the body is given to the person with back trouble for assessment in identifying:

- Where the pain is felt and when.
- What sensations there are in the back, arms and legs.

Figure drawings can be extremely useful in assessing information from the back sufferer and will often identify true signs from those of a malingerer.

DRIVING

See **cars**.

DRUGS

People with back pain can become addicted to or dependent on drugs which may be prescribed:

- For reducing inflammation in an **acute back**. (See **anti-inflammatory**.)
- For relaxing muscles which are in **spasm**. (See **painkillers**.)
- For counteracting **depression**. (See **anti-depressants**.)

Some painkillers and muscle relaxants may make you drowsy and less alert, so do not drive, as your concentration will be reduced. Drugs combined with alcohol will have adverse effects, and constipation and gastric upsets can also result from the overuse of certain drugs.

DURA

The inner lining or sheath, forming a fibrous skin or sleeve around the nerves in the spinal canal and around the nerve roots, is called the dura or dural sheath. (See **nervous system**.) It is extremely responsive to pressure and it is mobile from the top of the canal to the bottom. (See **compression**, **epidural injection**, **referred pain**.)

Inside this sheath, which extends into the brain as the dural membrane, is the cerebrospinal fluid which acts as a shock absorber for the **spinal cord** and **brain**. The dura thus forms an important barrier protecting the spinal cord.

DYES

The injection of various X-ray opaque dyes is used frequently to assist the **diagnosis** of back problems. Different types of dyes are used in special **X-rays** such as **myelograms** to show all the aspects of the back; the dye is injected into the dural sheath, is readily absorbed and provides very little adverse reaction. (See **dura**.)

DYNAMIC

Be dynamic – keep moving!

ELASTICITY

If **muscles** are not used and moved through their normal range regularly, there will be a loss of elasticity, the muscles will become tight, which will limit **joint** movement. Attempts to move the back will then cause tugging on the tightened muscles around the joints, with resulting pain.

Regular **activity** and specific **exercises** will keep the muscles flexible and maintain their elasticity.

'Exercise to keep elastic.'

ELECTRIC BLANKETS AND PADS

Warmth, when it is applied directly to the problem area, is a tried and tested remedy to relieve backache. Electrically heated products are now made specifically for the purpose of bringing instant relief; the blankets or pads are shaped to wrap around individual regions of the back, enveloping the aching area with gentle warmth. There is usually a choice of heat levels for maximum comfort and you should establish that the product has received a British Standards Institute approval. Regular checks to see that the blanket or pad has not become damaged are essential and the product should be carefully stored. Never leave the pad on for longer than 10 to 15 minutes at a time. (See **electrotherapy**.)

If you do not like using electricity, a hot water bottle or gel pack will provide similar warmth. (See **heat therapy**.)

ELECTROMYOGRAPHY

Electromyography (EMG) is an extremely helpful diagnostic procedure, used by qualified experienced physicians, which indicates whether surgery is necessary and in which area of the back. It determines exactly what is wrong with the spinal cord or individual nerve roots, distinguishing irritative from destructive damage to the nervous system, and whether a specific nerve is not transmitting messages to a muscle simply due to pressure. (See **compression**, **disc**, **nervous system**, **referred pain**.)

An electromyogram (EMG) detects and provides a record of nerve impulses to the muscles and the response of the muscles. Fine needles are inserted into the various muscles of the back, arms or legs in order to determine the site of the complaint, and they are attached by wires to a recording machine. A slight pricking and stinging sensation may be felt as the needles are inserted, but the tests usually last only a short time. The contractions are shown on a screen and recorded on a print out. The recognition of normal and abnormal traces from various muscles can then be used to diagnose nerve root damage from pressure, injury or disease.

ELECTROTHERAPY

Electrotherapy is not usually considered practical for home application as most equipment is designed for professional medical use, in which safety regulations have to be considered. For example, **ultrasound**, lasers, pulsed magnetic currents, **diathermy**, interferential therapy and **transcutaneous nerve stimulation** may all be employed in the treatment of back conditions by chartered physiotherapists.

However, electrical stimulation can be self-administered with a transcutaneous nerve stimulation; this will relieve pain, but you should be taught how to use it correctly by a registered qualified practitioner.

EMOTION

Emotions play a large part in everyday life. Psychological research has shown that pain can be intensified if you are angry, bored, insecure, depressed or have **stress** due to some other human behavioural problem. (See **anger**, **depression**.) Learn to know yourself emotionally, and try to understand whether you are dealing with physical or mental pain and whether you are using one to disguise the other.

ENDORPHINS

These morphine-like substances are generated naturally by the body to combat pain. Endorphins are released into the cerebrospinal fluid, and their production can be stimulated in a variety of ways such as by **acupuncture** and **transcutaneous nerve stimulation**, thereby avoiding the use of drugs.

ENERGY

Self-generating high-octane energy is the life force and the secret of looking after your back. In order to have mental and physical energy, you should have a balanced lifestyle. You cannot do everything, you are only a human being, and stress and strain which block physical and mental function, will stop your energy flow. You need lively motivation to stimulate the maximum number of nerve cells which will fire the energy in the maximum number of muscle fibres for good physical fitness.

What to do

- Decide what tasks are essential and limit the time you spend on non-essential activities.
- Make time to **relax** and rest; spend time with your family and friends.
- Delegate chores to the family or to others in the office.
- Take regular active **exercise** to increase your oxygen intake. This will improve the ability of your body to burn oxygen and calories.
- Keep sugar intake down to a minimum.
- Fight fat by taking exercise and altering your diet if necessary.

- Take contrast baths of hot and cold water to revive your circulation.
- Eat plenty of fruit and vegetables and take a supplement of **vitamins**.
- Have an active love life.
- Walk tall with good **posture** rather than moaning and groaning.
- Be positive – smile and enjoy life.

EPIDURAL ANAESTHESIA

The dural space between the spinal cord and vertebral column can be injected with local anaesthetic to numb the nerve fibres and therefore relieve pain. (See **dural sheath**, **injections**.) There are two sites for such injections, the caudal and **lumbar regions**. (See **cauda equina**.)

Epidural anaesthesia may be used for low back pain during childbirth or to numb the spinal cord against the pressure or friction being caused by a protruding **disc**.

EQUIPMENT

There is a great deal of equipment, from **beds** and **chairs** to **pillows** and lumbar **supports**, both cheap and expensive, to help back sufferers.

ERECTOR SPINAE MUSCLES

These **muscles** hold the back erect. They are not visible, but they provide the posterior support for the back. They work hard when **pushing** or **pulling** heavy weights, **bending** forwards and backwards, or when you hold the back very erect.

ERGOFORM CHAIR

See **chairs**.

ERGONOMICS

Ergonomics is the science that has evolved to reduce the friction between man and work. It is the study of the physical relationship between the worker and the work environment; for example, when seated to work, the height of the work surface in relation to the height of the chair should be comfortable, with both feet resting on the floor. The environment can then be planned for the activities involved, to ensure the best results, in the office, the factory or the home.

The application of ergonomic principles will produce greater efficiency for the same amount of effort, and as a spin off will prevent back problems. In an ideal situation, furniture, fitments throughout the house, and surfaces at work will be ergonomically designed to fit the individual's body and lifestyle, thereby preventing stress and strain on the back. (See **chairs**, **desks**, **house-work**, **kitchen**, **office**, **visual display unit**, **workplace**.)

- Plan your worktops so that they are the correct height for you in the kitchen, the bathroom, the garage and the greenhouse.
- Assess your workplace; for example, if you are a typist, is your chair at the right height for you?
- Learn to bend, lift and carry loads correctly. (See **carrying**, **lifting**.)

NOTE: If you want to invest in ergonomic furniture, make sure you go to a specialist shop where trained staff will understand your needs and take time to guide you in finding the right solution.

EXAMINATION

If you have to have a back examination from a doctor, a consultant, a chartered physiotherapist, an osteopath or any other medical practitioner, this is what happens.

- You will be asked to relax, having first undressed to your underwear.
- While you are sitting on the edge of the couch, reflexes will be tested at the knee and ankle with a light hammer to see if there is any **nerve** impairment.
- **Muscles** are tested, and you will be asked to lie on your back, raise each leg up, keeping the knee straight until you feel pain. This is known as the straight leg raising test, or SLR.
- Skin sensation is checked with a pin.
- Palpation movements are used on the back to detect signs of tenderness or **spasm**.
- Observations are made of your **posture**.
- All movements of the back such as **flexion**, **extension** and **rotation** are checked in the standing position, to see which produce pain and whether there is any increase or decrease in the natural **curves** of the back.

EXECUTIVE

The bad back of an executive in his or her office is usually due to:

- Poor seating and **desks**. (See **chairs**.)
- Poor lighting. (See **eyes**.)
- Lack of rest and **relaxation** causing tension and **stress**.
- Gripping the telephone tightly, looking at the VDU or reading the balance sheet!

Always consult a specialist shop for **ergonomic** office furniture, where trained staff will help you find the right solution.

EXERCISE

'Better to hunt in fields,
  for health unbought
Than see the doctor
  for a nauseous draught
The wise for cure on exercise depend
God never made his work, for man to mend.'
John Dryden, 1631-1700

Exercise should be fun. It aims to:

- Mobilise and strengthen the back, abdominal, bottom and thigh muscles in order to avoid problems.
- Build up general fitness, which will increase your self confidence.
- Help normal functional activities so that there is no fear in performing the movements.

Normal movements of the back

- Forwards or *flexion*.
- Backwards or *extension*.
- Sideways or side flexion.
- Turning or *rotation*.

Questions to ask yourself

Before starting on a long-term course of exercise, ask the following questions – they will help you decide what to do.

- Do you enjoy doing things on your own?
- If not, do you need company and discipline?
- Can you plan ahead and stick to the plan?
- Are you too busy to exercise properly?
- Do you want to involve the family?
- Are you restricted by a small child?
- Are you overweight, over 40 or unfit?
- Should you only choose a few exercises so you do not get bored or tired?

Basic rules for exercise

- Warm up before you start.
- Do exercises as regularly as cleaning your teeth.
- Make time each day.
- Relax between each exercise and at the end. (See *relaxation*.)
- If it hurts do not do it.
- Do not get overtired.
- To start with, three or four exercises are quite enough, done three or four times each. Progress slowly to five exercises

done five times and then ten exercises done ten times.
- Control and concentrate on each exercise, making them rhythmical and smooth.
- Take up an activity when you feel fit.
- Cool off and wind down, putting on more clothing after an exercise routine.

Exercise programmes

You may need exercise to relieve **pain**, prevent **stiffness** and/or build up strength.

There are many exercise programmes, from hard driving aerobics, aimed at muscle burn, to low-impact exercise, where one foot is nearly always on the ground. You should choose an individual programme especially fashioned and tailored for your back, and perform regular amounts of modest enjoyable exercise. If you need help, ask a therapist. The following entries detail some exercises.

- *Abdominal exercises*.
- *Balance*.
- *Breathing exercises*.
- *Calf muscles*.
- *Extension*.
- *Flexion*.
- *Groin*.
- *Hamstring*.
- *Knees*.
- *Mobilising exercises*.
- *Neck*.
- *Pain*.
- *Pelvic tilt*.
- *Relaxation*.

NOTE AND WARNING: Ask your doctor if you are in doubt about doing exercises.

EXTENSION

When the back arches or extends backwards from the mid-line, it is called extension. The bony structure of the *vertebrae* only allows a slight degree of extension as the range is limited by the spines of the vertebrae. The movement should never be forced, as compression of the **facet joints** will result and the anterior longitudinal **ligament** will become overstretched. (See **compression**, **disc**.)

Many people who sit or stand continually in the forward flexed position can benefit from extension exercises for the lower back.

Extension exercise

Also known as a McKenzie extension exercise.

- Lie face down on the floor in a position similar to a press up, with your hands flat on the floor, level with your shoulders.

  Place your elbows under the shoulders and push up, arching the upper back until you can lean on your forearms. Hold for the count of five and lower slowly. Repeat five times. Try not to hunch your shoulders.

- A progression of this exercise uses the same starting position. Then push up your arms to arch or extend the back, but keep your hips on the floor. As you lift the head and shoulders off the floor, keep the chin tucked in. Hold for the count of five, and then gently and slowly lower to the starting position. Relax. Repeat five times if you can, trying to arch a little more each time.

EYES

Have your eyes tested regularly, as poor eyesight can cause back problems – peering at a blackboard in school or straining to see the road ahead when driving will result in lower back **strain** and **neck** ache, as will bending and stretching the neck to peer at incorrectly placed VDU screens. (See **cars**, **visual display unit**.)

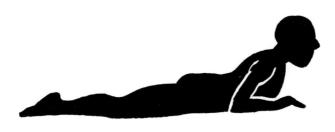

Extension exercise

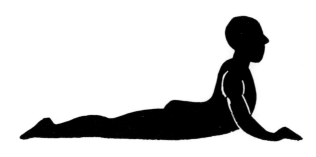

Progression of extension exercise

FACETECTOMY

This term describes the surgical removal of a **facet joint**.

FACET JOINTS

The **vertebrae** are joined to each other by two small facet **joints** at the back part of the body of the vertebrae. They are synovial **joints**.

FAINTING

Dizziness and fainting can sometimes occur when you stand still for a long time. This is due to the lack of muscle movement in the back and legs, and the subsequent slowing down of the blood being pumped around the body back to the brain. (See **circulation**.)

FASCIA

The connective tissue found all over the body surrounding the more delicate structures is called the fascia. It is thick and tough, consisting of bundles of white fibrous tissue. It forms the superficial fascia in the upper back and neck. The deep fascia tends to be thinner, and there are three layers in the **lumbar region**. The fascia forms the sheaths of **muscles** and, in some areas of the back, contains granular **fat**.

FAT

Fat is laid down between the layers of **fascia**, just below the skin as well as deeper. If injury should occur to the fascia, a small globule of fat may push through the stretched tissue. When the fascia is no longer stretched, the fatty globule can become pinched which can cause pain in the tissues.

'Be fit not fat!'

FATIGUE

The most common form of fatigue is the 'tired housewife syndrome'. Young and middle-aged women should reflect carefully if boredom, tiredness, unhappiness or disappointment are the cause of fatigue and a bad back. It may be necessary to streamline the kitchen and have everything at the right level for your back, to make household tasks easier so you avoid continual **twisting**, **bending** and overstretching in the home.

All of us have to do some boring tasks in everyday life, so a change in routine or taking up a new activity or sport can often alleviate fatigue. A day off, a holiday, rest or relaxation for a short period, and a good night's sleep will all help. (See **ergonomics**, **executive**, **housework**.)

FEET

Since standing and walking are necessary everyday actions, great respect should be given to the feet to avoid problems, for example in growing children, during pregnancy and in later life.

Most people's feet are perfect when they are born. However, three in four adults have some kind of foot problem and this can affect the back, so good foot care is essential.

- Go barefoot as much as possible. Feel the difference in your back and your **balance**. (See **babies**.)
- High heels put too much weight on the front of the foot, squash the toes and narrow the base for **standing**. (See **posture**.) The **pelvic tilt** is altered and an increased **lordosis** can result. The back suffers strain in order to keep an upright posture.
- 'Negative' heeled shoes are also a hazard.
- Wear flexible soft **shoes** with thick soles to prevent **jarring**. Leather is best for uppers

with soft crepe soles and laces, with a buckle or velcro fastening to hold the heel in place.

- A fastening over the instep stops the foot sliding forwards and the toes can grasp the ground better, so **walking** improves.
- Foot exercises can help walking and therefore help the back generally.
- Foot rollers help **circulation** in the foot and **ankles** and improve muscle mobility.

At the end of a hard day, don't just get off your feet – give them a treat with contrast baths of hot and cold water for 10 minutes then a quick **massage**. (See **chiropodist**, **podiatrist**.)

FELDENKRAIS

This technique was develped by Doctor Moshe Feldenkrais who was born in Russia in 1904. Dr Feldenkrais was a physicist and engineer, as well as a judo expert. The method teaches people to move in an easier, more efficient manner by promoting good posture which in turn reduces **fatigue** and **stress**.

The objectives of the technique are:

- Increased awareness and discipline.
- Enhanced economy of movement.
- Improved functioning in everyday life.

The method is taught either in group classes or on a one-to-one basis, with awareness through movement, so that your regular routine is enhanced for the benefit of your back, neck and shoulders. See the Where To Get Help section at the end of the book.

FIBROSITIS

Fibrositis means **inflammation** in the fibres of the **muscles**. The most common areas of fibrositis are the muscles of the **neck** and upper **shoulders**, and the outer part of the **buttocks**.

Fibrositis describes the painful tender pressure points which are often called **nodules**, 'knobs',

or **trigger points** since they trigger off pain and discomfort when they are pressed. The musculo-skeletal hardness and stiffness, which is often worse in the morning and causes fatigue, is now being called fibromyalgia in America. It has been found to affect women more often than men.

- Have localised treatment for the tender fibres of the muscles. (See **acute back**, **physiotherapy**, **massage**.)
- Change your working **posture**, as often fibrositis is caused by holding your head forwards in a tense position. (See **ergono-mics**, **workplace**.)
- Do a gentle programme of **exercises**.

FIRST AID

This can be necessary for a sudden problem if you have a fall or a severe injury to the back.

In an emergency get medical help IM-MEDIATELY. Don't move the patient until the ambulance or medical help arrives. (See also **acute back**.)

FITNESS

If you are fit you will reduce the likelihood of hurting your back, and ensure a rapid return to normal everyday life if you should suffer an injury. Remember that moderate **exercise** taken over a long period is far better for health and fitness than indulging in enthusiastic extremes which can lead to tiredness and injury.

Combine a good **diet** with regular exercise. A crash diet will not work, since you need the calorie intake from food to make the energy that is necessary for fitness.

FLEXFIT

The Flexfit lumbosacral support has been designed by Spencer of Banbury. It was develo-ped as a lightweight elasticised alternative to traditional steel back corsets, which tended to restrict movement and were often uncomfortable.

The principle of the support, while limiting back movement and assisting the **abdominal muscles** during an acute phase, also allows flexibility as the muscles improve in strength. It ensures support at all times, especially in the forward **bending** motion because the flexible pad moulds itself to your shape and stays with you as you bend. It is completely unobtrusive under clothing and is easily washable. (See **corsets**.)

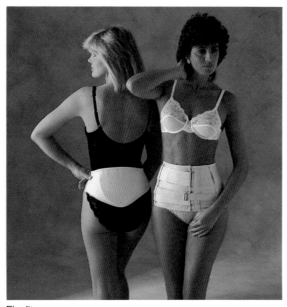

Flexfit supports

FLEXION

When the neck and lower back bend forwards from the mid-line, it is called flexion and is a difficult movement to perform when the back hurts. (See **pain**.) It is important to maintain flexion in the back and not to allow the **muscles** to become stiff and rigid. The **hips** also take part in flexion and can be exercised at the same time.

Forward flexion

Sit on the edge of a firm chair. Bend forwards, sliding your hands down your legs to touch the floor – just flex forwards as far as is comfortable for your back. Hold for a count of five. Return to the starting position, uncurling slowly, and relax for a count for five. Repeat five times.

Side flexion

This movement is away from the mid-line and is limited in range by the vertebral bodies and **discs**.

Stand with your feet apart, arms by your sides, head erect and the chin tucked in. Bend first to the left and then to the right, keeping the head in line with the trunk. Stretch the left hand towards the left knee for the count of five and then repeat to the other side in a slow rhythmical fashion.

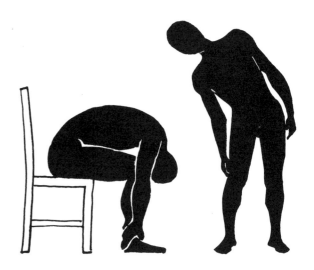

Forward flexion   Side flexion

FOETAL POSITION

A very comfortable **position** when there is **pain** in the lower back.

FOOD

Without becoming a bore about food and drink, be aware of what is good for your body and make sure you have information about the dietary values of food. (See **diet**, **vitamins**.)

FOOTBALL

Football is a much better contact **sport** for the back than rugby, although back injuries may occur when overstretching to head a ball, **jarring** the spine on hard ground when jumping or running, and in a **twisting** fall when tackling an opponent.

FORAMEN

A foramen is the opening found between two adjoining **vertebrae** which allows the passage of the nerve root and blood vessels.

FRACTURE

A fracture is a broken bone. It may be an avulsion fracture, in which a small piece of bone becomes broken away from a vertebrae due to continual stress or an injury, or it may be a compression fracture of the back, which is much more serious. **X-rays** will confirm whether or not there is a fracture.

FUN

Having a bad back is no fun. If you become tense and worry over work, the family, finance or competitive sport, life will not be fun. (See **emotions**, **stress**.) Put things into perspective if you want to avoid backache and have fun.

FURNITURE

Well-designed furniture is extremely important for the back as it can PREVENT back problems. Take time to choose the right furniture for your individual use, both in the home and at the workplace. The right heights and width of the various pieces of furniture are essential and you should learn how to use them correctly. (See **beds**, **chairs**, **desk**, **ergonomics**, **tables**.)

There is a video cassette available called *Mind Your Back* which shows you how to use items of furniture. (See under Suggested Further Reading, at the end of the book, for details.)

FUSION

Spinal fusion is the surgical joining of one **vertebra** to another using techniques such as bone graft, screws and wires. Such an operation will be necessary if abnormal and excessive movement has caused permanent **instability** in one region of the back which cannot be improved by strengthening exercises of the **muscles**.

During a fusion, due to the cutting of the tissues, **inflammation** occurs which may result in the formation of **adhesions**. Also, since the fusion will cause loss of movement in one region of the back, **stress** will occur elsewhere as a compensatory effect since another region has to work overtime, causing other **joints** to become irritated and inflamed. New bony growth occurs as a result of a fusion and this can cause pressure on nerves and blood vessels, entrapping them and resulting in referred problems. (See **compression**, **referred pain**.)

For these reasons surgical fusion should not be undertaken lightly but only after careful and lengthy discussions with the consultant and after everything else has failed to solve the problem and the pain.

FUTON

The futon is a Japanese **mattress** which has been in use for the last 4,000 years. It provides a firm and comfortable **bed**, enabling the back to settle in its natural position during sleep. It can be rolled up by day on to a slotted wooden base to become a sofa.

GARDENING

'Oh Adam was a gardener, and God who made him sees
That half a proper gardener's work is done upon his knees.'

Rudyard Kipling, 1865-1936

Gardening is a popular outdoor activity which puts demands on the back and can be hard work. The over-ambitious who rush out and dig the garden on the first day of spring are asking for back trouble. Before gardening, especially in cold weather, warm up your muscles first. **Squatting**, **kneeling**, **bending** and **stretching** exercises will help your back for the tasks ahead. The Chartered Society of Physiotherapy will provide a leaflet on how to care for your back when gardening. See Where to Get Help.

Wear **clothing** that is comfortable and keeps you warm in cold weather. Well-fitting **shoes** and gardening gloves will help you to grip and lift correctly.

Tools

- Make sure the implement suits your height and build. It should not be too heavy and the handles should be long enough for you to avoid stooping. (See **bending**.)
- Wheelbarrows should not be overloaded as **pushing** will become difficult. You should keep the handles close to the body.
- The incorrect use of flymowers can cause swinging of the body from the waist and **twisting** of the back. Use your feet to change direction and keep your body in line with the mower.
- Store tools at the right height for you and in an orderly fashion, so there is no strain in getting them in and out of a shed.
- Use powered tools whenever possible, providing they are not too heavy for you and do not vibrate too vigorously. (See **jarring**, **vibration**.)
- Long-handled tools are available to make hoeing and pruning easier.

What to do

- Take the strain with the legs rather than the

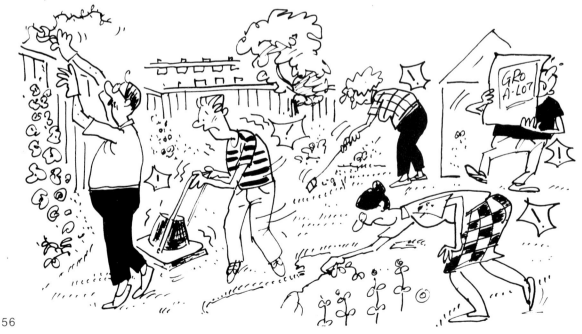

back. Strong thigh and bottom muscles are essential.

- Keep the back straight and don't stoop or lean over a spade or fork.
- Change your working position frequently and try to maintain the natural lumbar curve of your back.
- Use long-handled tools.
- Shovel and lift small amounts of earth each time, especially if the soil is heavy and wet.
- Avoid overdoing it and STOP if an ache develops in the back.
- If your back is really stiff convert most of the garden to a lawn or paved patio with only a manageable area for plants and flowers.
- Stock the garden with perennials, to cut down on the annual work.
- Mulch beds to keep the weeds down and use a long-handled hoe or fork.
- Have tubs and pots at waist level where possible, and raise the flowerbeds. (See **ergonomics**.)
- Install garden taps and an automatic watering system at the right height.
- Use a trolley or get help if you need to carry a bag of peat or fertiliser, and observe the rules for **lifting**.
- Don't bend down or over-stretch to pull the odd weed or root of a tree out of the ground.

Let your arms and legs take the strain. Crouch down and bend your **knees**.

- Kneel on a padded stool or kneeler, or squat to plant or weed.
- Don't stay in one position for too long.
- Make sure the **abdominal muscles** are not sagging when you are planting and weeding.

Gardening is a satisfying creative pastime especially for the elderly, but you must think how to do it, plan carefully and have a rest when you have finished.

GLUTEUS MAXIMUS AND MINIMUS

These are the **muscles** of the **bottom** or buttocks which you use when you squeeze your bottom. They are used for balancing the **pelvis** and **hips,** for **standing** and **walking**, and for **extension** of the back.

GOLF

Golf is a very popular enjoyable **sport**, but has a high incidence of back problems, usually due to poor technique, plus a lot of bending and

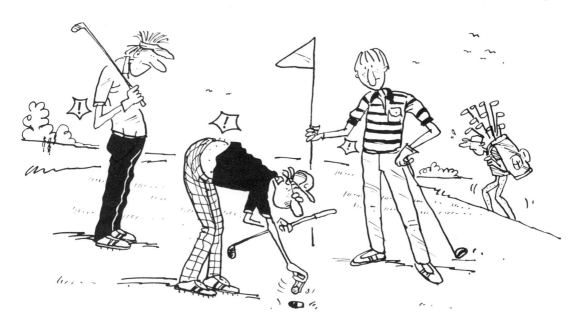

crouching. Very tall and very short people can have problems and should have clubs specially made for them. *Jarring* the spine with a poor shot on hard ground will cause pain.

What to do

- If you have an acute attack of back pain, STOP immediately. (See *acute back*.)
- Don't rush back to the game as you will probably have another episode. Start slowly and gradually build up to full fitness by doing specific *exercises*.
- Bend down correctly to get the ball out of the hole. (See *bending*.)
- Only carry a few clubs, and if you use a trolley push it rather than *twisting* the back to pull it. (See *carrying*, *pushing*.)
- Squat and do some knee bends while waiting on the tee rather than standing around with a sagging tummy and an exaggerated *lumbar* curve. (See *abdominal muscles*, *knees*, *lordosis*, *squatting*.)
- It may be necessary to change your swing, so consult the golf professional or watch yourself on a video.
- Wear a *corset* if your abdominal and back muscles are weak.
- Keep the back warm.

GRAVITY

Man stands upright, so *muscles* have to overcome the forces of gravity. It is therefore extremely important that they are all strong enough to support the back in a balanced *posture* in order to avoid falling forwards or tipping sideways as a result of the pull of gravity.

Gravity can be used as a form of traction for the back. (See *inversion therapy*.)

GRIP

It is essential to learn how to grip and handle loads and equipment correctly in order to avoid problems for the back when *lifting*. Hoists and *slings* can be used if there are no hooks or handles on the load. The fingers should be curled into the handle or hook; if the fingers are straight, they will tire easily and the extra *strain* will be taken through the arms, the shoulders, the neck and the back.

GROIN

Exercises to stretch the groin will improve the mobility of the lower back and the inside thigh muscles.

Stretching exercise

Sit on the floor with your legs apart, your knees bent and the soles of the feet touching – the frog position. Hold your ankles, resting your elbows on your knees. Bend forward towards the feet, curling the back. Hold for a count of five and then uncurl slowly. Repeat, stretching forward a little further each time.

You will find this exercise difficult if you have tight hamstring muscles.

GYM

Many people join a gym in order to exercise using the specialised equipment. It is often more enjoyable to exercise in the company of other people in a gym, and your back will certainly benefit from the regular exercise. Home gyms are now available, but when purchasing such equipment you should ensure that it has been recognised and it is reliable. (See *Norsk Sequence Training Machines*, *Tunturi* and gym equipment in Where to Get Help at the back of the book for details of distributors.)

GYNAECOLOGY

This is the treatment of disorders of the female reproductive organs. Such disorders can cause pain in the lower back; for example, frequent heavy periods, a large retroverted uterus or a prolapsed womb can cause a dull dragging pain in the lower back. Surgery, with perhaps removal of the womb by a hysterectomy, may be necessary.

If you think you have any gynaecological disorders see your doctor or a gynaecologist immediately.

HABIT

'How use doth breed a habit in man!'
Two Gentlemen of Verona,
William Shakespeare, 1564-1616

Back problems can arise as a direct result of bad habits. (See **backache**, **crossed legs**, **posture**.) So avoid bad habits if you wish to prevent back problems.

HAMSTRINGS

This group of muscles is attached to the **pelvis** near the top of the thigh at one end and runs down the back of the thigh to the knee, inserting in the lower leg. The muscles bend the **knees** and ensure flexibility of the **hips**, thereby assisting the back in **flexion**. In full flexion they are stretched so that the pelvis is brought forwards to a horizontal plane.

Test for tight hamstrings

In a relaxed fashion, bend the head and neck gently forwards, slide your hands down the front of the legs and let your arms drop to the floor if possible. Touch the floor, keeping the knees straight. Do not bounce to the floor, as it can cause severe pain or a tear in a muscle tendon. Measure the distance between the fingertips and the floor. Use this measurement to evaluate flexibility after stretching the hamstrings.
NOTE: Uncurl slowly, tightening your bottom and tummy muscles until you have a good erect posture again.

Hamstring stretching exercise

Sit on the floor with your legs stretched out in front of you. Then tuck the right foot up so that it is against the opposite knee.

Bend your trunk towards your left knee and reach with your hands to grasp your left ankle or foot. Hold for five and relax. Repeat with the right leg. Do not bounce or strain; just gently stretch the hamstrings.

HANGING

Since the time of Hippocrates in 500 BC, hanging has been a useful method of relieving **back pain** and pressure on the **discs**. By hanging from a door, wooden bar or the banisters and allowing the legs to relax, the weight of the legs will exert a **traction** force on the back. (See **inversion therapy**.)

Hanging from a door

- Take care to hang near the hinges of the door so you do not pull it down.
- Jam the door open so it does not swing shut and trap your fingers.
- Grip the top of the door, having padded it with a soft towel, then slowly bend the knees keeping the toes touching the floor.
- Keep the arms straight, but do not lock the elbows; if they are braced, muscles in the back will contract.

HEADACHES

Headaches are one of the major causes of human suffering. They are often associated with back problems as a result of tension and muscle spasm in the **neck**. If you suffer from headaches, you need to ask yourself what is the cause of the headache, and what can be done to get rid of the problem and the pain.

Find the cause

- Is it due to a muscle **spasm** from a draught or an injury?

- Are you tense due to **anxiety**, **depression** or **anger**?
- Do you have poor **posture**?
- Do you have high or low blood pressure or is your **circulation** altered in any way by heat or cold?
- Do you suffer from migraines or an allergy?
- Have you an eye, ear, nose, or throat infection or tooth problem?
- Is the cause a hangover?
- Are you constipated?

What to do

- **Aspirin**, paracetamol or another **analgesic** drug may help you.
- Have treatment for muscle spasm, especially if it's in the upper back and neck muscles.
- Practise **relaxation** and rest with the eyes closed and the head and back well supported with **pillows**.
- Try and have regular sleep for a maximum of eight hours and check the position of your pillows.
- Eat a balanced **diet**.
- Exercise regularly by **walking** or **cycling**. However, if you swim it may cause a headache since the position of the head with the neck held in too much **extension** above the water can lead to problems. (See **swimming**.)
- Do not smoke, and avoid smoke filled atmospheres.
- Learn to express your feelings in a direct but non-aggressive manner – get it off your chest or receive counselling. (See **emotions**.)
- **Massage** any painful nodules in the neck and upper **shoulder** region.
- Have **mobilisations** and **manipulation** after X-rays if there is a mechanical problem.
- Correction of posture of the head and back is essential.
- Wear a **collar** if the headache has been caused by an injury to the neck.

NOTE: See your doctor if you cannot get rid of your headaches. And always seek professional advice if sinusitis, bad influenza or more serious conditions such as meningitis, concussion or a head injury are the cause of the headaches.

Migraine headaches

True migraine headaches are often associated with nausea and vomiting, and vision problems usually precede these symptoms due to constriction and then relaxation of the blood vessels on one side of the head only. Research is showing that feverfew, a member of the chrysanthemum family, suppresses the hormone serotonin which has been found to be a cause of migraine. **Transcutaneous nerve stimulation** may also help.

HEALTH AND SAFETY AT WORK

It is important that hazards for the back are avoided at the place where you work. The Health and Safety at Work Act (1974) states that 'it is the duty of employers to ensure so far as is reasonably practicable, the health, safety and welfare at work of all his employees', but it is also your responsibility. (See **workplace**.)

HEAT THERAPY

This is a useful method of relieving the muscle **spasm** which often causes back pain. Notice how animals sit in sunny spots or float in warm pools.

Heat should generally be applied at least twice a day for no longer than 15–20 minutes at a time, as stiffness from lack of movement will result if you lie too long under the sun or a lamp. Deep heat can also be produced in the tissues by a medical practitioner using **electrotherapy**.

Heat is not a cure for back pain, but it affords temporary relief by increasing the **circulation** in the inflamed area prior to other techniques such as *massage* and *mobilisation*. Never use a fierce heat or use heat after you have had a linament rub.

Some sources of heat

- Hot water – showers and spa therapy.
- Hot water bottle.
- Hot towels which have been steamed.
- Sunshine.
- *Infra-red* heat lamps.
- *Electric blankets and pads*.

SPENCO HOT WRAP

The Spenco Hot Wrap is a flexible pack containing Hydroflex gel. It is soothing and convenient to use for *acute back* conditions, providing *heat therapy*. The Hot Wrap can be heated in a microwave oven and it then retains its heat for the recommended time for therapy.

HEELS

Tight heel tendons, the Achilles tendons, sometimes can cause back pain especially if high heels have been worn for any length of time. *Stretching* exercises will be helpful. (See *calf muscles*, *feet*.)

HELLERWORK

See *massage*.

HELP

There is a Where To Seek Help section at the end of this book. However, this book was written to help you to help yourself.

- Keep your *muscles* moving and in good tone.
- Try not to wear heels that alter your individual *balance*. (See *shoes*.)
- *Rest* if your back hurts.

- Buy a good firm *bed*.
- Have a *car* seat that fits your back.
- Change your *position* frequently.
- Try not to sit when you can stand or walk about. (See *walking*.)
- Have a long *mirror* in the house so you can check your *posture* daily.
- Learn a method of *relaxation*.
- Smile and you will feel better.

HERBAL MEDICINE

Not only herbs but weeds, roots, shrubs, trees and flowers have been used for thousands of years, with beneficial effects for certain problems. For example, various herbal creams or oils are used in aromatherapy *massage* to treat muscle spasm and aches in the back.

HEREDITY

Sometimes abnormalities in the back can be inherited from parents or grandparents. (See *abnormal*.) These are usually noted at birth or in the growing child.

While no two backs are ever alike, it is wise to seek specialist advice if there is a history of back problems in the family. Hopefully any symptoms can be discovered and the cause eliminated at an early stage. Be observant and constantly watch the growing stages of your children. (See *observations*.)

HERNIATED DISC

The protrusion of the nucleus of the *disc* which squeezes out through an opening in the annulus, pinching nerves in the back, is known as a herniated disc.

HIPS

The hip *joints* and the movements of the hip *muscles* are vital to smooth back function.

When seated the hip joints function best if they are opened out to approximately 135 degrees, but sitting on a typical upright straight chair fixes the hips at an angle of 90 degrees or less. When you move forwards over a desk this angle is compressed further and the pressure on the hip joints is usually relieved by collapsing the low back. This compresses the abdominal region and places an abnormal load on the back structures. It is therefore important to see that you choose a chair that is correct in design for your back and hip angles. (See **chairs**.)

There are five groups of muscles supporting the hip: hip extensors, hip flexors, hip abductors, hip adductors and hip rotators. They act together to provide **balance** and stability for the back for such actions as **standing** on one leg. Any damage to any of these groups will reflect on the back as the alignment of **posture** will be disturbed. **Walking**, **cycling** and **swimming** will exercise all of these muscles.

HOISTS

Hoists are compact manoeuvrable items of equipment which can be used in both the hospital and the home, removing the need for aides, nurses and the family to carry out heavy **lifting**. They are used in conjunction with **slings**.

HOLIDAYS

Holidays can be a great tonic for a bad back, especially if the problem is due to overuse of the back from hard work, tension or severe **fatigue**. But if you are going away from home for a holiday, make sure you find out the following.

- If you are staying at a hotel in a strange **bed**, is it suitable for your back?
- Are suitable seats available for **air travel** and long distance driving? (See **cars**.)
- If you are swimming or doing some other activity during the holiday, make sure you are fit enough, and have warmed up first. (See **exercise**, **sport**.)

- Will you expose the back to sudden extremes of **temperature**, such as lying on an airbed in cold water after sunbathing? If so, you will return from your holiday with a bad back!

Holidays should be a period of rest and **relaxation**.

HOLLOW BACK

An expression to describe the excessive curve in the lower back. (See **curves**, **lordosis**, **lumbar region**.)

HOMEOPATHY

Homeopathy comes from the Greek word *homoio*, meaning like or similar, and *pathos* meaning suffering; together they imply 'like suffering'.

The principles of homeopathy were laid down by the German physician Samuel Hahnemann in 1811, but were first suggested by Hippocrates who lived in 500 BC. The diagnosis and treatment are based on the whole body and the theory that 'like can cure like', with an emphasis on a person's history and habits. For example, if a substance causes anxiety when given to a healthy person, the same substance will cure someone suffering from anxiety.

A single remedy is selected from a list of up to about 3,000 substances, on the basis that it will cause symptoms that most closely match those you describe and will fit in with your personal history. The remedies, which are given in minute amounts, are derived from plants, minerals and animal extracts.

Homeopathy can be used to treat back conditions such as a stiff **neck**, a strained lower back, **tension** and **arthritis**. See the Where To Get Help section at the end of the book.

HORMONE REPLACEMENT THERAPY

See *osteoporosis*.

HORSE RIDING

See *riding*.

HOSPITAL

In certain cases a doctor or specialist will recommend that you should go into hospital for an operation or for much the same treatment as you may be having at home.

- Bed rest will be total, with no getting up to answer the door, the telephone, or put out the cat.
- Everything that is being done at home – bed rest, *traction*, and the administration of drugs – can often be better accomplished in a hospital. (See *acute back*, *drugs*.)
- Special tests, such as *CAT scans* which may be necessary to establish the cause of the back problem, can be easily carried out. (See *electromyography*.)
- Professionally trained nurses, doctors and chartered physiotherapists will be on constant call.

Hospitalisation is an expense, but if, by leaving home for a few days for proper treatment, recovery from back pain results, then it may be worthwhile. If on the other hand being in hospital leads to depression and other psychological complaints, it is better to stay at home.

HOUSEWORK

If you wish to avoid back problems, be practical and realistic about housework. Get the family to help you if you have *acute back* pain, and let the dust settle.

'A bit of dirt never hurt.'

Tips for housework

- Dish washers can be a real back hazard due to the height of the machine and the frequent *bending* necessary to load and remove the dishes and cutlery. It is worth considering a model that is put up on the draining board if your back is very bad.
- Use long-handled feather dusters and upright vacuum cleaners. Kneel down where possible to avoid too much intensive bending and stooping to dust furniture or when you clean out the fire grate. (See *kneeling*.)
- Standing at the ironing board can be another hazard for the back, and many people prefer to sit on a suitable *chair* with the ironing board lowered to the correct height. (See *ergonomics*, *posture*.) If you have to stand ironing for prolonged periods, relieve some of the pressure on the back by elevating one foot on to a small stool.
- Have a long-handled milk bottle holder, or squat to lift the milk bottles.
- Try and always have two people to empty a full litter bin or trash can, or have a trolley for the dustbin. (See *lifting*.)
- Ovens, fridges and freezers should all be at eye level to avoid bending or stooping.
- Try and have heavy objects at working height so you do not have to over-stretch or reach up to lift them down. If you have to lift something down from an overhead cupboard, make sure you do it safely. Use steps or stand on two chairs on a non slip surface and take off your shoes; have a stable base and *balance* your back, tightening your tummy muscles as you lift and lower the object from the cupboard. (See *abdominal muscles*.)
- While working at the kitchen sink, have your feet slightly apart to give you a stable base.

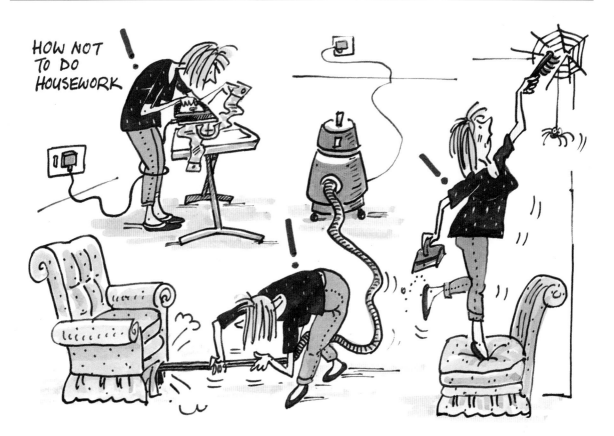

Put a bowl on the draining board if the sink is too low and work at this level. (See *ergonomics*.) Have the taps moved to the side of the sink with levers fitted to them to prevent reaching across the sink and *twisting* and straining the back. Stand on a small platform if you are short. Intermittent *stretching* over the sink will relieve backache.

- Front-loading washing machines, especially in a narrow confined space can cause back strain from twisting and bending. Buy a top loader if you have a really bad back. However, if you do have a front-loading machine, sitting or *kneeling* on the floor is better than twisting.
- Vacuuming is one of the most hazardous occupations in the house, especially if you have a canister tubular vacuum with a hose and nozzle that you pull across the floor behind you. The upright vacuum cleaners are much better for a bad back – they are easier to push although they cannot get in all the nooks and crannies.

When vacuuming, stand upright with the knees slightly bent and use short strokes, avoiding unnecessary *bending*. (See *posture, pushing and pulling, standing*.)

HYDROTHERAPY

The enjoyment of warm water has been favoured for many centuries and is still used in many European countries, where spas are an important industry and 'taking the waters' has traditionally been part of medicine. *Chronic back* sufferers have been particularly receptive to this form of therapy. Among other advantages, the effects of exercise in water for chronic back pain, using water assistance and resistance, are extremely valuable for strengthening the muscles of the back and for general fitness. (See *swimming*.)

HYPERMOBILITY

If *joints* are too mobile, it is called hypermobility. You can be hypermobile in several joints. However, a back that is hypermobile in one or two joints is often caused by adjacent joints having poor mobility or *hypomobility*.

HYPNOTHERAPY

Hypnotherapy can help someone with *chronic back pain* when orthodox medical diagnosis is unable to establish a cause. The hypnotherapist will alter your state of consciousness inducing a deep physical *relaxation*, relieving painful symptoms, so you are open to positive suggestions about your physical and mental state.

HYPOCHONDRIA

Hypochondriacs rarely complain of back pain. It is too common and too boring!

HYPOMOBILITY

When there is reduced mobility in the *joints*, it is known as hypomobility.

HYSTERECTOMY

See *gynaecology*.

ICE

See *cold therapy*.

ILIA

The pelvic girdle is formed from two large bones, the ilia, which meet at the front at the symphysis pubis by way of the pubic bones. They articulate at the back with the sacrum, forming the *sacro-iliac joints*. (See *pelvis*.)

INACTIVITY

'For too much rest itself becomes a pain.'
Homer – eighth century BC

Muscles are weakened by inactivity which will leave them vulnerable to injury. Find a prog-ramme of *exercises* which suit you, and become active.

Don't be lazy. Your back will suffer.

INDUSTRY

Over the years there has been an increasing desire to prevent back pain in industry. Occupa-tional medicine has looked carefully at the relationships between workloads and the inci-dence of pain, especially in the lower back, both in the manual labourer and the sedentary worker. It has been observed, for example, that typists have a higher incidence of back pain than coal miners, and disc injury is less common amongst manual labourers than sedentary workers. Many employers now have personnel responsible for *biomechanics* and *ergonomics* in the *work-place*.

This concentration on occupational health should:

- Reduce *bending*.
- Reduce *twisting*.
- Reduce reaching.
- Reduce *lifting* and lowering force.
- Reduce the weight of objects.
- Reduce *pushing and pulling*.
- Reduce *carrying*.
- Reduce the use of incorrect *furniture*.

Conveyor belts, hydraulic lifts, slides, chutes, hoists, slings and well-designed furniture all help at work, but age, the monotony of the task and other factors should be also taken into considera-tion.

INFLAMMATION

Inflammation is a reaction in the tissues that have been hurt due to:

- A mechanical irritation of a joint.
- A muscle injury or tear.
- An infection.
- A chemical reaction.

Extra fluid is formed at the site of inflammation, which may be acute or chronic.

Acute inflammation

Immediate swelling occurs as extra fluid accumu-lates in the injured tissues, the swelling varying from severe to microscopic, depending on the nature of the damage. The fluid is sticky and is composed of blood and clear *lymph*. *Ad-hesions* may occur due to the inflammation, which will restrict movement resulting in stiffness and pain. (See *acute back*.)

Chronic inflammation

The fluid which has wept into the joints or tissues becomes slowly thickened and hardened with time, resulting in the formation of fibrous tissue, which further restricts movement. Adhesions may occur, and *muscles* can become wasted. (See *chronic back*, *fibrositis*.)

INFRA-RED HEAT

An infra-red heat lamp may be recommended for relieving muscle **spasm** and increasing the **circulation** in the painful area of the back. Lamps can be purchased from large chemists or electrical stores. You should read the instruction leaflet carefully for any precautions, and check that the bulb is up to the required standard. Take care not to fall asleep under the lamp.

A dry heat can be very soothing, but it is not a cure. An electric heating pad or hot water bottle will produce almost the same effect as an infra-red lamp. (See **electric blankets and pads**, **heat therapy**.)

INJECTIONS

There are several types of injections to help back pain, which are used for specific purposes when the back is too tender to respond to physical treatment.
NOTE: The value of injections will vary, depending on the individual and the medical practitioner who is giving them, so always consult a fully qualified person every time.

Epidural injection

See **epidural anaesthesia**. If you have an epidural it is important to ask what procedure you will receive; ask your doctor to explain exactly what happens and what the possible contraindications may be. You should decide for yourself if you want it, especially during **childbirth**, and not necessarily have it thrust you on.

You may have pain for several days after an epidural, and if this pain persists, seek medical advice.

Scelerosing injections

These injections are given by medical practitioners, usually into a weak **ligament** of the back. The injection results in a local **inflammation**, leading to the formation of **adhesions** and causing a firming up and hardening of the tissues. Ask what happens and if there are any real benefits.

Hydrocortisone injections

These injections are given in small amounts to tender areas to relieve pain and inflammation. Ask your doctor to explain the possible side-effects.

Lignocaine injections

When other conservative methods have been unsuccessful, an injection of dilute lignocaine is given by a specialist to interrupt the pain reflex arc, followed by a single forceful manipulation to ensure that a full range of movement is obtained.

Chymopapane injections

Chymopapane is an enzyme derived from the tropical fruit, papaya. It is used extensively as an injection, under X-ray control, into the centre of the **disc** as an alternative to surgery.

There can be allergic reactions to the drug, and the chemical shrinkage of the disc leading to disc degeneration can cause further back pain. Research is now showing that complications are being reduced, so this method may be used more widely in the future.

INJURY

Injury to the back can take place throughout life. When giving a history to the doctor or any other medical practitioner it is important to try and recall any injury you may have had in the past. (See **diagnosis**, **questions**.) A bad fall, a skiing accident or a road traffic accident as a teenager might not have worried you at the time but can cause real back problems when you are older.

Often, though, you know when you have damaged yourself because the pain is usually instantaneous, such as in a twisting **sprain**, a stretched torn muscle or a **strain** from bending over and feeling that something in the back 'goes'. Severe injury to the back will always need hospitalisation.

INSTABILITY

When unnatural movement keeps occurring in one area of the back, it is considered to be an unstable segment of the spine. Something usually causes the instability, such as a bad fall from a horse or when skiing, repeated manipulations over a period of time, pregnancy or childbirth.

- Wear a **corset** for heavy jobs.
- Avoid repeated **manipulation**.
- Do strengthening **exercises**.
- Modify **shopping** expeditions. (See **carrying**.)
- Change your **position** frequently.
- Avoid **standing** for too long.
- Don't become **overweight**.

If the problem persists and there is pain and deformity, it may become necessary to have surgery to correct it with a spinal **fusion**, in order to make the back more stable.

INTERVERTEBRAL

This means between the **vertebrae**. (See **anatomy**.) The **discs** are often described as intervertebral discs.

INVERSION THERAPY

This is the modern name for the ancient practice of hanging upside down, which was advocated by Hippocrates in 500 BC. Due to ingenious new equipment, gravity controlled **traction** in the upside down or inverted position, is now relatively simple. A tilting board offers you total control on how quickly you wish to invert and how far you wish to go.

Reversing gravity for a few minutes every day has the following benefits:

- It relieves pressure on the **discs**.
- It relieves **compression** on nerve roots.
- It stimulates the **circulation** and aids lymphatic drainage.
- It stretches **muscles**.
- It relieves **tension** and realigns the back.

Standing on your head in a yoga position has some of the same effects but you need to be extremely fit, with strong neck muscles.

Contraindications

- **Acute back** conditions.
- High or low blood pressure, angina and heart conditions.
- Damaged lower limb **joints** or **ligaments**.
- Artificial joints.
- Menstruation and pregnancy.

There are other side effects and contraindications, so check with your doctor before using any kind of inversion equipment.

IRONING

See **housework**.

ISOMETRIC EXERCISES

The word isometric comes from two Greek words, *isos* meaning equal and *metria* meaning measurer. In these **exercises** the **muscle** tension changes but the length of the muscle remains the same.

These exercises are the safest and most effective way to start building up muscle strength after an **acute back** episode. A position is adopted and the position is held by a muscular contraction which is working in moderation and not for maximum power. The muscles are strengthened by increasing the bulk of the muscle fibres, as the contractions are done against the resistive force of a similar process in the opposing group of muscles. As no joint movement takes place, it will not aggravate an acute situation.

ISOTONIC EXERCISES

This comes from the Greek words *isos*, equal, and *tonos*, tension. In these **exercises** the muscle tension stays the same but the length of the fibres change, moving the **joints** with each muscle contraction.

JACUZZI

Taking the baths was very popular with the Romans; today a modern development, the whirlpool bath, invented by Roy Jacuzzi in California in 1968, is a lovely way of treating your own back. A jet of warm water directed at a stiff sore area is painful initially, but it increases the **circulation** in the region, eventually relaxes the muscles, helps mobility and is very pleasant. **Hydrotherapy** and spa baths are being more widely used at health hydros today, while the jacuzzi is becoming more popular at home.

JAMMING

When the facet **joints** of the **vertebrae** become locked it is sometimes called jamming. It is not advisable to have any thrusting **manipulation** for this as it will weaken the **ligaments** further, resulting in stretched unstable structures.

See the Where To Get Help section at the end of the book for registered qualified practitioners who may be able to help.

JARRING

Jarring occurs when a trivial movement, such as stepping down a deeper step than you expected, sneezing, a violent cough, a car or truck ride on a rough road or a bad aircraft landing, jars your back. The muscles are caught off guard and a quick agonising pain is felt in the back.

What to do

- Learn to brace your **abdominal muscles** and be aware of situations so you counter-act the effects of jarring.

- Wear a support **corset** or **collar** if you know your back is weak and you have a history of jarring incidents.
- Do exercises for the abdominal muscles.
- Rest for 24 hours after a severe jarring, and use **heat therapy** or **cold therapy**.

JET LAG

The effects of long-distance **air travel** may cause back problems due to tense muscles from hours of sitting still. It can be alleviated by **isometric exercises**, eating light meals, avoiding alcohol and drinking plenty of non-carbonated water. Try to rest and sleep as much as possible, for at least 12 hours, after a long tiring flight, especially if there is a big change in the time factor.

JOGGING

If you have recurrent low **backache** you should not jog; jogging can jar the back as you take each step, due to the effect of the body weight. (See **biomechanics**.)

When jogging, the body is slightly ahead of the centre of gravity, with an increased lumbar curve. **Jarring** through the foot, up to the knees, the hips and then the back, especially on tarmac roads and uneven surfaces where no spring in the foot can occur, is hard on the back. (See **vibration**.)

If you enjoy jogging:

- Select a good pair of running **shoes** from one of the recognised manufacturers. They should be lightweight, shock absorbing, with thick spongy soles, especially at the heel. Never wear gym shoes.
- Do **warming up** exercises, especially for the **hamstrings** and the **knee** muscles.
- Wear plenty of clothes if the temperature is low. You can always take them off and tie them round your waist.

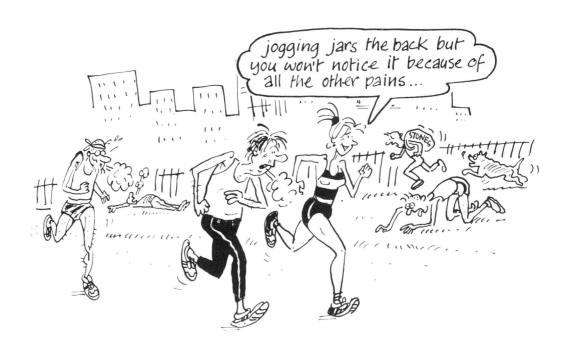

- Jog on a rebounder at home in bad weather, and on a smooth grassy surface or athletic track outside. (See **rebounding**.)
- Start slowly and build up endurance gradually.

And if you have a weak back, don't jog – walk or swim instead.

JOINTS

Where one **bone** or **cartilage** meets another there is a joint.

Intervertebral cartilage

With the **vertebrae**, a pad of cartilage lies between the bone surfaces of the vertebral bodies and there is a fibrous capsule to hold the bones and cartilage in place. The cartilages of such joints, the intervertebral **discs**, also act as shock absorbers between the bodies of the vertebrae.

As you get older, and with the stresses and strains of everyday life, ageing in the joints occurs. **Degeneration** can start in your 20s but is more common in the 40–50 age group.

Pivot joint

The first two **cervical** vertebrae form a pivot joint which allows the head to turn in a wide range. This joint is very vulnerable, and **headaches** can result if movement is not controlled. (See **atlas**, **axis**, **neck**.)

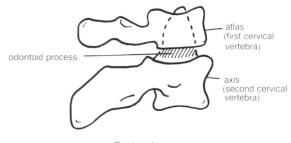

Pivot joint

Facet joints

Two small joints called facet joints link the bones together at the back part of the body of the vertebrae. They are **synovial** joints and permit slight gliding movements, allowing **flexion** and **extension** of the back but preventing sideways movement and **rotation**. They have an enclosing capsule, ligaments and a very rich nerve supply. The joints are connected to the weight-bearing body of a vertebra by bony bridges, the laminae, which form a continuous bony canal to protect the **spinal cord**.

If you bend, lift or twist with a weak back, the facet joints can become jammed together, so flexibility is lost and movement becomes difficult and painful. (See **bending**, **jamming**, **lifting**, **twisting**.)

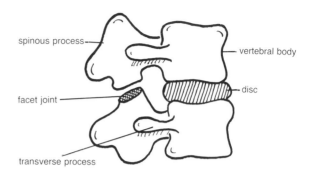

Position of facet joint

JUMPING

See **parachuting**.

KIDNEYS

Stones in the kidneys can cause back pain. If you think you have kidney problems, seek medical help immediately.

KINESIOLOGY

Kinesiology is the study of movement and the anatomical changes that take place as a result, while applied kinesiology is a healing method dealing with functional health disturbances as opposed to pathological disorders.

A series of musculoskeletal tests using energy balancing techniques was developed chiefly by Doctor George Goodheart, an American from Detroit. Tom McLurg Anderson developed advanced ideas on kinetics and body function, publishing his theories in 1951, many of which are incorporated into back classes today. He observed that most muscle **spasm** is not primary but secondary to opposing muscle weakness.

This method of treatment, which is also useful as a diagnostic tool, can prevent back problems by balancing the energy flow throughout the body, helping **posture**, **stress** and movement.

KITCHENS

Most people suffer from bad backs at some stage while working in the kitchen. It is essential to have your kitchen ergonomically designed and well lit if you are going to avoid problems. (See **ergonomics**, **housework**.)

KNEELING

Many people, when they have a bad back, find kneeling on all fours is a very comfortable position from which to start gentle **mobilising exercise**. When making the **bed** or weeding the garden, kneeling will help you avoid straining your back. (See **gardening**.)

KNEES

Since the knees are used in conjunction with the back, **hips** and **feet** for many activities, especially **lifting**, it is important that the knee muscles are strong. The quadriceps femoris is the name given to the group of four muscles on the front of the thigh which extend the knee joint and control **flexion**.

Quadriceps exercise

Sit on a firm surface with the back well supported and the legs stretched out in front. Pull the foot of the right leg up at the ankle, pushing the knee down to the floor or bed and tightening the thigh muscle. Hold for five and relax. Repeat with the other leg. Keep the leg as straight as possible and practise this exercise frequently.

A progression of the exercise is to flex the foot of the right leg up at the ankle, keeping the knee straight and the thigh muscles tight. Lift the leg up a few centimetres from the floor, hold, then slowly lower and relax. Repeat with the other leg. Once the knees are stronger, small weights can be added at the ankle.

KNOTTED MUSCLES

'Knotted' is a metaphorical term used to describe what you feel in a group of **muscles**, and is also sometimes used by medical practitioners to describe the muscle tone felt when you are undergoing treatment. In fact muscles cannot 'knot' as they are attached at each end but, since it is a way of describing a feeling, it is a useful expression.

KYPHOSIS

Kyphosis describes the forward curve of the thoracic spine. If it becomes exaggerated the resulting round back is sometimes called a 'dowager's hump' or 'The Hunchback of Notre Dame'. It may be just a bad postural habit, but it can become fixed and permanent.

Some causes of permanent fixed kyphosis are:

- *Heredity*.
- *Scheuermann's disease*.
- An abnormality from childhood.
- A disease such as *ankylosing spondylitis*.
- Osteoporosis.

What to do

Watch growing children for signs of kyphosis, poor *posture* and vague *backache*.

- Have a mattress which supports the thoracic curve when sleeping. (See *beds*.)
- Have gentle mobilising and strengthening *exercises* for *extension* of the back.
- Learn postural re-education by attending a back class or having *Alexander Technique* sessions. (See *back school*, *posture*.)
- Go *swimming*. The breaststroke is a helpful movement.
- Learn to lift correctly. (See *lifting*.)

Don't droop – the tiara will fall in the soup.
NOTE: Never have a manipulation if kyphosis is due to disease.

LABOMATIC WORKING CHAIR

See **chairs**.

LABORATORY TESTS

Tests may be necessary if back pain is prolonged or very severe. They are important for diagnosing conditions of the back such as **ankylosing spondylitis** and rheumatoid **arthritis**. (See **blood tests**.)

LAMINA

The flattened part of bone on either side of the arch of a **vertebra** is called a lamina.

LAMINECTOMY

Laminectomy involves the surgical removal of some of the bony **lamina** of the **vertebra** at the back of the spinal canal. This relieves pressure on the **spinal cord** and nerves, and any obstructing bits of **disc** can be removed to prevent pressure on the nerve root. (See **compression**.)

This operation is necessary when there has been unbearable pain over a period of time and the pain has radiated into the legs too. There may be numbness, pins and needles, muscle wasting and loss of power in the back and legs. Bladder and bowel sensations may also be impaired. A laminectomy is a major operation and will only be done by a surgeon after extensive tests such as **X-rays**, an **electromyelogram**, a **CAT scan** and a period of conservative treatment including **rest**, **traction**, **manipulation** and other pain relieving procedures.

What happens

- You will start walking 2–3 days after the operation, according to your surgeon's wishes.
- You will be in **hospital** approximately 10–14 days.
- You will be able to start gentle duties after three weeks.
- You will be taught correct **lifting** and handling techniques.
- You will not be able to do any heavy work for at least 3–6 months.
- You may have to wear a **corset** for a time after surgery until your muscles have regained their strength.

The back will be quite stable after the operation, but **scar tissue** may cause further painful problems. It is therefore wise to have a good talk with the surgeon before undergoing this operation as the use of **anti-inflammatory** drugs and an easier lifestyle may be an alternative, with surgery as a last resort. However, if you undergo surgery, ask what rehabilitation procedures are available and join the local branch of the National Back Pain Association. See Where To Get Help section at the end of the book.

LEGS

The best **exercises** for the back usually involve the use of the legs as well, once any **acute back** pain has disappeared.

Walking is best.

LESION

This word refers to **adhesions** of spinal joints, and is often used by osteopaths and other manipulators to describe this symptom.

LEVERS

Levers are basic to the understanding of movement and are used every day. The system of leverage is very helpful in trying to understand how your back works in various activities and how weight and force affect the movements of the back. (See **biomechanics**.)

A lever is normally assumed to be in a state of equilibrium, though in practice the forces acting on it may produce movements which are centred about a point called the fulcrum. In general, two forces act, the effort and the load. The effort is the force applied to hold the load in equilibrium; for example, the muscular effort needed to lift a weight.

A booklet is available from the National Back Pain Association which explains the principles of levers. (See Where to Get Help at the back of the book.) Learning these principles will help avoid back problems during such tasks as chopping wood, pushing a wheelbarrow or casting a fly when fishing.

LIFTING

Lifting is one of the major causes of back pain. No object is a safe load – they are all a risk, but heavy loads are more of a hazard. If a load feels heavy or looks too unwieldy and bulky, get help.

Rules for lifting

- Mentally prepare for lifting like an Olympic weightlifter. Concentrate on the object that needs lifting, so you can do it safely. For example, can the load be divided into two lighter loads? Can it be taken in stages? Can a mechanical pulley, **sling** or **trolley** help?
- Check your **clothing**. Safe lifting means carrying things close to your body, so it is

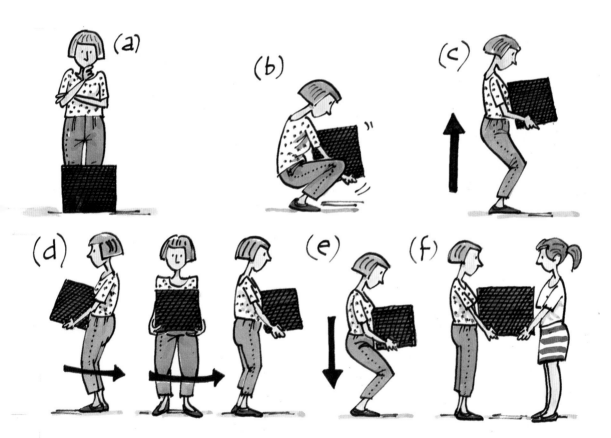

Lifting

foolish to wear clothes with loose flaps, or trousers that are too tight to bend your knees. Wear **shoes** with non-slip soles and low heels, and strong gloves if an object is slippery.

- Check the area to see that there are no obstructions like a balustrade, a greasy or slippery wet floor, or a high back to a car boot.
- Work out how to **grip** and handle the weight. Where are you going to put your hands?
- Place your **feet** correctly. It is safer to stand close to the object, with your feet apart, facing the way you want to go, with one foot in front of the other. If the feet are together you will have a small unstable base.
- Bend the **hips** and **knees**, keeping the back straight and the **shoulders** level, facing the same way as the **pelvis**. Squat down, getting a firm grip on the load, using the whole of the hand, not just the finger tips. Hold the arms close to the body with the elbows tucked in. (See **bending**, **squatting**.)
- Raise the object up by straightening your knees. If your **abdominal muscles** do not tighten automatically when you lift the load, learn to brace them just before you lift.
- Beware of **bending** sideways as you lift, and avoid **twisting** and turning. If you have to change direction during the lift, turn your feet as well as your body. Remember this when lifting a bucket of water if the tap is in an awkward position.
- Lift the object quickly and smoothly, with a slightly swinging motion, keeping the load close to your body throughout the lift.
- Do not hold the load any longer than is necessary, and always put it down carefully by squatting again. Put the load down again immediately if it is too heavy for you.
- Better still, if a load is too heavy, do NOT move it. Seek help and plan how two of you can move the object. Wait until your partner comes home or ask the supermarket assistant or a porter to help you.

'Practice makes perfect.'

Notes and warnings

- **Pulling** is generally less stressful than pushing.
- It is easier to lift a load when it is raised, even a few inches off the floor. Between the knee and hip is the best height for efficient lifting. (See **ergonomics**.)
- If you are tired it is unwise to lift. (See **fatigue**.)
- Lift loads in stages. Stop and have a rest between stages.
- Heavy manual lifting can be taught in a **back school** class, and you will benefit if you are a farmer, a builder or a nurse and have to handle sacks, barrels, patients or any other heavy weights.

LIGAMENTS

Ligaments act as guy ropes, along with the **muscles**, to support the central backbone. (See **anatomy**.) Ligaments are strong tough bands of white fibrous tissue which connect one bone to another. They stabilise the back, controlling and guiding movement. The ligaments tense or stiffen when you move forwards and relax as you bend backwards, thus preventing the bones from tipping sideways. Ligaments are slightly elastic and flexible, but when they are stretched beyond the limit of their elasticity they tear and are painful. If they are stretched for prolonged periods they become elongated, rather like overstretched knicker elastic, and can eventually ping or snap, resulting in disaster!

Sprained and strained ligaments as a result of poor **posture** at work or a sudden forceful effort are a common cause of back pain. They heal slowly and not very well as they do not have a rich blood supply. (See **sprain**, **strain**.) The **sacroiliac** ligaments are especially vulnerable in pregnant women, since during **childbirth** an enzyme is released into the ligaments, increasing their elasticity. (See **pregnancy**.)

NOTE: **Standing** in a shop all day, going round an art gallery, or queuing for long periods can strain the ligaments of the **feet**, causing you to stand badly which will result in backache.

Longitudinal ligaments

There is an anterior (front) and posterior (rear) longitudinal ligament running the length of the back, lining the vertebral bodies. These wide long ligaments also constitute the outer layer of the annulus of each **disc**. The posterior ligament has a rich nerve supply and can be easily damaged if the **abdominal muscles** and back muscles are weak.

LINIMENTS

People often equate liniment with horses. However, rubs or sprays can be very effective in the short term as they produce a reaction in the skin and superficial tissues, increasing the **circulation** and helping underlying muscles, thus relieving **spasm** and **inflammation**. Ask your pharmacist to recommend a good liniment for **massage**.

LOCKING

This is when the **facet joints** become locked or jammed. (See **jamming**.)

LORDOSIS

Lordosis describes the curve formed in the **lumbar region** and **cervical region** of the back. When this is exaggerated or excessive in the low back, it is called a sway back or hollow back. You can be born with this weakness in the lumbar **vertebrae**, but it is usually due to:

- Poor **posture**, with the body weight being carried too far backwards.
- Weak **abdominal muscles** which cause the tissues in the back to shorten, showing a marked curve or lordosis, and the tummy to become more protuberant.
- A marked **kyphosis** which affects the **neck**.
- Poorly designed seating. (See **chairs**, **ergonomics**.)

What to do

- Do regular **pelvic tilt** and **abdominal exercises** to increase the stability of the **lumbar region**.
- Mobilise the lumbar region by doing **flexion** exercises.
- Correct your posture and make sure your chin is tucked in all the time.
- Wear a **corset** if it provides support when you are in pain.
- Invest in a good **bed**, **chair** and **car** seat to fit your individual lumbar **curve**.
- A back **support** will help you cope with poor seating in restaurants, theatres and cinemas.

LOW BACK PAIN

See **backache**, **degeneration**, **lumbar region**, **pain**, **rotation**.

LUGGAGE

See **carrying**, **lifting**, **suitcases**.

LUMBAGO

An expression used to describe pain in the **lumbar region**. The muscles in the area seize up and go into **spasm**, which is extremely painful. Lumbago is usually caused by bad postural habits, **draughts** or poor **furniture**. (See **acute back**, **backache**, **posture**, **spasm**.)

LUMBAR PUNCTURE

This describes the entry of a long needle into the dural sheath in the **lumbar region** to withdraw spinal fluid or inject a dye for tests. (See **dura**.)

LUMBAR REGION

The lumbar region is the lower part of the back and consists of five large **vertebrae** sitting on the **sacrum** below the thoracic spine. (See **anatomy**.) They are numbered, top to bottom, L1 to L5. They are larger than the vertebrae above as they have to provide greater support and bear the body weight. When you are seated the load on the individual vertebra can be as much as 200 lb per sq. inch.

The lumbar region is the most vulnerable area of the back as it does most of the work. Over the age of 50, when **degeneration** has occurred, care should be taken with the movements in this region. (See **lordosis**, **lumbago**, **pelvic tilt**, **posture**.)

LUNGS

If there is an infection in the lungs, there may also be pain in the ribs and the back. See a doctor promptly. (See **bronchitis**, **thoracic region**.)

LYING DOWN

See **positions**.

LYMPH

Lymph is the colourless alkaline fluid circulating through the lymphatic system of the body. When damage to the back occurs, lymph oozes into the tissues as part of the process of **inflammation**. (See **circulation**.)

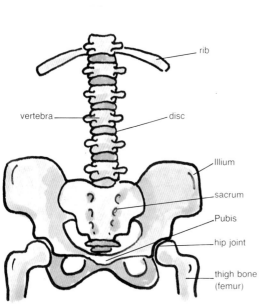

Lumbar region: front view

rib

vertebra — disc

Illium

sacrum

Pubis

hip joint

thigh bone (femur)

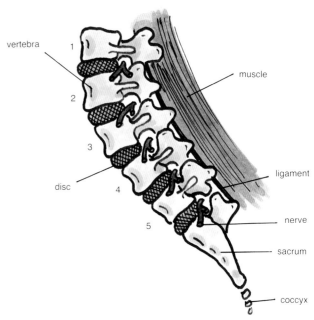

Lumbar region: side view

vertebra   1

2

3

disc   4

5

muscle

ligament

nerve

sacrum

coccyx

McKENZIE

Robin McKenzie, a New Zealand physiotherapist, was born in Auckland in 1931. He developed techniques for treating the back and neck which are now used by physiotherapists worldwide. His specialised treatment of back disorders has demonstrated that active exercises for the back will resolve problems. (See **extension**.) He has also designed a Lumbar and Cervical Roll for use in the curves of the back, and a Night Roll. (See **supports**.)

In 1982 the McKenzie Institute was formed to provide an orderly development of education and research into his methods. He has written two best-selling books on the subject of self help for back treatment, *Treat Your Own Back* and *Treat Your Own Neck*, which have helped countless back and neck pain sufferers around the world. See Suggested Further Reading at the end of the book.

MAGNETIC RESONANCE IMAGING

Magnetic resonance imaging (MRI), like a **CAT scan**, provides an image of the whole body. It is a very sophisticated technique that measures magnetic fields within the body. It enables neurologists and surgeons to establish internal **disc** disruption and **degeneration**.

MAITLAND

Geoffrey Maitland, an Australian physiotherapist, has developed certain manual techniques, known as Maitland **mobilisations**, for mobilising the back and other **joints**. They are gentle rhythmical passive pressure movements that are performed manually by a therapist to increase the movement within the limit of the normal range of the **facet joints**, preventing them from becoming stiff. The mobilisations are made without any thrusting action so that there is only gentle stretching of the **ligaments**.

MANDAL

Doctor Aage Mandal, a Danish surgeon and physician, having suffered from back pain himself in 1967, was concerned that sitting had caused a dramatic increase in back problems. Having observed the patterns of behaviour of children on school seating, Mandal developed a **chair** with a seat that tilts forwards. He tried to reduce the strain and pain of sitting by developing a seat with a forward tilt of 15 degrees and an adjustable angle, to reduce the tilt and friction and so prevent any feeling of sliding down. (See **Balans**.) Doctor Mandal is famous for his book *The Seated Man – Homo Sedens*. (See the Suggested Further Reading section at the end of the book.)

MANIPULATION

Manipulation has been used for centuries as a treatment for the relief of back pain. When an individual **vertebra** is manipulated, the mobility of movement in the back improves due to the controlled force that removes the restrictions in the **joints**. An accurate diagnosis should always be established by a qualified medical practitioner before you have a manipulation.

Having chosen the vertebra and the direction of movement after an exact **examination** and **diagnosis**, the manipulator will use the hands quickly and deftly to 'crack', 'pop', 'unlock', or 'thrust' – all expressions used to describe the movements which remove the restrictions in the joints. As a result, the associated problems of limited movement, muscle spasm and stiffness will be relieved in the back. If after two or three treatments there is no improvement, then manipulation is not right for your back and you should seek further advice so that **ligaments** do not become over-stretched and the back unstable.

It is important to have a programme of **mobilising exercises** and postural re-education to prevent stiffness or fixation occurring again after the manipulation. (See **posture**.) You may feel slightly below par the day following a manipulation due to the after-effects, so ask your practitioner to give you advice on a post-manipulative regime. (See **chiropractor**, **osteopath**, **physiotherapist**.)

There are contraindications for manipulation in conditions such as **ankylosing spondylitis**, acute rheumatoid **arthritis**, **spondyloliesthesis** and **osteoporosis**.

Cervical manipulation

Care should be taken in the **neck** region during **cervical** manipulation because of the **spinal cord** travelling in the narrow spinal canal and the proximity of the **brain**. (See **anatomy**.) Numbness and loss of movement could result if manipulation is performed incorrectly. Always consult a registered qualified practitioner, who should make sure an **X-ray** of the neck is taken before performing a manipulation.

Manipulation under anaesthesia

If your back is too painful for a practitioner to manipulate, it may be necessary to have a manipulation under anaesthesia, which will be performed by a surgeon and followed by a regime of mobilising exercises taught by a physio-therapist to maintain the full range of movement.

MASSAGE

The value of touch as a natural means of therapy has been recognised since ancient times. It is extremely beneficial for the relief of muscle **spasm** in the back, while even simple stroking of the back induces a wonderful soothing effect, producing deep **relaxation**. However, massage on its own cannot cure back pain, and sometimes it can even aggravate it, for example in conditions such as **sciatica** or acute **arthritis**.

Effects of massage

- Loosening up the muscle spasm and tightness in the tissues.
- Increasing the blood supply to the **muscles**, producing a warm glow.
- Producing a soothing and relaxing effect on the body.
- Relieving *tension* and breaking down **nodules**.
- Helping backache during **childbirth**.
- Releasing pent up **emotions**.

Aromatherapy

This aims to treat the whole person by using essential oils which are massaged into the skin. The oils are extracted from the aromatic part of plants and flowers. Although their effect is not a recognised scientific treatment for back problems, the subtle powers of the oils may soothe away stress and tension, while a general improvement in circulation occurs with the application of the back massage techniques.

Connective tissue massage

Connective tissue or **fascia** is widely distributed throughout the back. This important **massage** technique stimulates the autonomic **nervous system** and improves **circulation** by rolling the skin and underlying tissues in the fingers. It breaks down **adhesions**, relieves muscle **spasm** and tension, and promotes general **relaxation**.

Hellerwork

Hellerwork, named after Joseph Heller, an aerospace engineer, evolved in 1978. It is practised in the United States of America and is now becoming fashionable in the United Kingdom. It is a series of sessions of deep tissue massage based on Rolfing, which with movement education is designed to realign the back and release stress and tension.

Rolfing

This technique was developed by Ida Rolf in the 1930s. It consists of deep massage to realign the body in its proper posture. The body is manipulated and massaged so that the mind and emotions are freed from any 'blocks', and the body can retain a healthy natural posture. In 1976, Joseph Heller became the first president of the Rolf Institute.

MATTRESSES

See *beds*.

MEDITATION

Back sufferers with chronic muscle *spasm* and who are generally anxious and tense will benefit from meditation or autogenic training, a form of self hypnosis. It is necessary to learn initially from a qualified teacher or doctor. (See *hypnotherapy*, *yoga*.)

MENOPAUSE

Osteoporosis may occur in the bones of the back during menopause and progressively afterwards. Hormone replacement therapy (HRT) is now becoming more widely used at this stage, and there is much on-going research into menopause. Ask your doctor or a gynaecologist whether the treatment is suitable for you as they will know about current research and methods of treatment.

MENSTRUATION

See *periods*.

MERIDIANS

This is the name given to the pathways or channels of energy flow in the body. (See *acupuncture*.)

MIGRAINE

See *headaches*.

MILITARY POSTURE

See *posture*.

MIRRORS

Learning how to create a good *posture* should be part of everyday life. A long mirror, or even two of them at right angles, is essential. It is especially helpful when correcting and teaching children.

Vanity is not a bad thing if it is going to promote an elegant good posture in *standing* and *walking*. Check yourself in a mirror frequently.

'Look good – feel good.'

MOBILISATIONS

See *Maitland*.

MOBILISING EXERCISES

Active mobilising exercises should be practised daily, as soon as they can be comfortably tolerated, after an injury in order to prevent *muscle stiffness* and wasting and to maintain a full range of movement in the *joints*.

Rocking

Lie on your back with your knees bent at a comfortable angle of about 45 degrees, knees slightly apart and your feet on the floor. Support your head and neck with a pillow and place your arms loosely by your sides.

Holding the *pelvic tilt* position, slowly bring one knee up to your chest, grasping the knee below the kneecap. Rock gently for a count of five, hold for five then relax. Repeat with the other

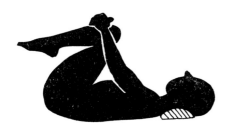

leg, and then hug both legs and rock them. However, if the pain increases after two or three rocks, stop the rocking exercise.

Rolling

The starting position is as for the rocking exercise above. Then, keeping your knees together, roll your legs gently over to the right, keeping your left shoulder on the floor. Hold for five, then return to the starting position. Now lower to the other side and hold. Repeat five times.

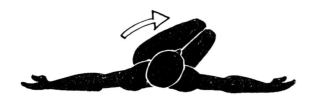

Arching and hollowing

Kneel on all fours, with the hands directly under the shoulders and the knees slightly apart so you have a stable base.

Arch your back into a curved round position, with your head tucked in between your arms, tightening your tummy muscles. Hold for a count of five. Now gradually sag, hollowing the back, and raise your head to look ahead. Control the

sagging movement, allowing the tummy muscles to relax.

If you have a headache or neckache, this exercise is not for you.

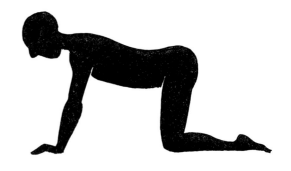

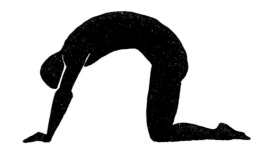

MORNING STIFFNESS

See *stiffness.*

MUSCLES

Muscles are composed of tissue whose cells have the ability to contract and relax. Muscles work both actively and passively, but in conjunction with each other, to perform specific movements, so that as one group contracts causing movement, another group relaxes allowing that movement. The muscles are attached to bones by *tendons* or *fascia*. There are 140 muscles attached to the framework of the backbone, the major functions of which are to produce movement, to balance the body against the forces of gravity, to protect and support the back, the **nervous system** and the internal organs and constantly adapt to your needs.

If you neglect your muscles, they will waste rapidly which will cause back problems. For example, as you bend over a desk or typewriter, muscles are called on to maintain body stability, and the longer they remain in this sustained contracted state, the more likely they are to become saturated with their own waste products. These waste products accumulate during the unaccustomed effort and exertion that prevents muscles from relaxing and effectively locks them into a state of tension; stressed muscles are weak and useless.

The low back muscles are the most significant in the **posture** of the back for, along with the tummy muscles, they hold the pelvis in the right position. When they lack strength, the pelvis tilts forwards and as a result the lower back arches and the tummy protrudes, and the body loses poise and grace. (See **pelvic tilt**.)

Self discipline is required if you are to use your muscles efficiently and effectively. Normal activities such as **walking**, **running** and **lifting** keep the back muscles in good **tone**, without any need for particular exercises. If your muscles have wasted specific exercises will help providing they do not cause any pain. They should not be too vigorous, as if you have back problems they will only cause further damage so it is wise to exercise little and often. The ideal situation is to exercise initially in water. (See **exercise**, **swimming**.)

Some of the important muscles used in the movement of the back are:

- The abdominal muscles. (See pages 1–2.)
- The bottom muscles. (See page 23.)
- The calf muscles. (See page 26.)
- The hamstrings. (See page 60.)
- The hip muscles. (See pages 62–63.)
- The knee muscles. (See page 74.)
- The neck muscles. (See pages 86–87.)
- The thigh muscles. (See page 127.)

MYELOGRAM

This is a special investigatory test which may be necessary to discover if there is possibly a prolapsed **disc**. A dye is injected which will show the shape of the **spinal canal** and the site of a damaged disc or a **tumour**. Once the dye has been injected, the back is **X-rayed** to determine whether surgery is necessary.

NACHEMSON

Professor Alf Nachemson, a Swedish orthopaedic specialist, has done much research to prove that **sitting** exerts more pressure on the spine than **standing**. His scientific evidence, which is recognised worldwide, shows that some motion of the back and regular **exercises** will benefit people with spinal problems. Clinical studies, bio-engineering studies and studies in other disciplines relevant to the back are continually being explored and researched in his department of orthopaedics in Sweden. (See Suggested Further Reading.)

NATUROPATHY

Naturopathy is an alternative therapy which may be of general benefit for back problems. This method of healing aims to eliminate disease by building up the body's own defences and self-healing powers and then removing toxins that have accumulated through stress, faulty **diet** or bad habits. Dietary changes, **hydrotherapy**, **relaxation** and manipulative techniques are all used by a naturopath.

NECK

The neck is made up of seven cervical **vertebrae**, numbered C1 to C7, which support the head. (See **anatomy, cervical region**.) The vertebrae are small and are held in place by an arrangement of 32 complex **muscles**.

The main functions of the neck are:

- To support the head and the structures within it, particularly the **brain**.
- To allow the head to move through 180 degrees from side to side, to bend forwards,

backwards, and to rotate by means of the pivot **joint** at the **atlas** and **axis**, C1 and C2. This wide range of movement, and the lack of surrounding protective structures like the ribs, make the neck the most vulnerable region of the back.

- To protect the **spinal cord**, which travels from the brain down the back to the **sacrum**. (See **nervous system**.)

Common neck problems

- Bad **posture**.
- Cervical **spondylosis**.
- **Fibrositis**.
- **Headaches**.
- **Neuralgia**.
- **Osteoarthrosis**.
- **Rheumatism**.
- **Whiplash** or wry neck.

Tight neck muscles

If your neck muscles are sore or tight you should rest, lying down, fully supporting the head and neck. (See **pillows, supports**.) Try **relaxation** techniques, and wear a neck **collar** if you have an injury or if you have to work or travel.

Have treatment to mobilise the neck; this may include **heat therapy, ultrasound** and **Maitland** mobilisations. Apply **massage** by learning the following techniques.

- Keeping the shoulders relaxed, place the little fingers at the base of the skull and position the rest of your fingers down the neck so that they rest at the base of the neck. Relax the hands. Using a kneading motion, work the fingers up and down the neck, working out from a central line.
- Keeping the shoulders relaxed, place the hands on the top of the back with the little fingers on either side of the base of the neck. Gently knead the neck from the base outwards and down to the shoulders. Return to the base of the neck and repeat.

Neck exercises

The following will exercise your neck and correct your **posture**. You should learn to distinguish between discomfort and pain when you are doing these exercises. Think carefully about the movements as you do them – they are all simple.

Sit in a good upright position on a firm chair, or stand to do these exercises, but make sure your **abdominal muscles** are pulled in, the **shoulders** are level and the head is straight with the chin tucked in.

Look straight ahead, pull the chin in and stretch your neck. Stretch up at the crown of your head and feel the distance between the shoulders and ears getting longer.

- Drop the chin slowly on to the chest, bringing it towards the notch between the collarbones. Hold for ten and return to the starting position.

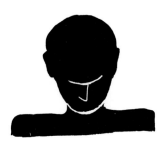

- Tilt the head to one side, bringing the ear towards the shoulder. Keep the shoulders still. Hold for ten and relax. Repeat on the other side.
- Tilt the head back just enough so you can see the ceiling. Hold for five and return to the starting position. Repeat.
  NOTE: Never snap the head backwards, causing a jerk and the neck to hyper-extend.
- Slowly turn the head to one side, trying to look over your shoulder to the point of full stretch – 45 degrees approximately, although it can be more. Hold for ten and return to the centre. Repeat on the other side.

Neck and head retraction
This exercise is extremely important since it helps postural pain which results from sitting over schoolbooks, office work, or driving the car.

Sit in a good upright position on a firm chair, or stand with the shoulders level and the arms relaxed by your sides.

Looking straight ahead, pull your chin in, straightening the neck so you stretch. Putting the tip of a finger on the crown of your head and

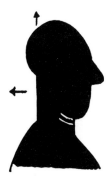

pushing upwards sometimes helps the feel of the exercise. Keeping this position, slowly raise and lower the shoulders. You can also roll the shoulders backwards, keeping the head and neck in the retracted position.

Note and warning

See a doctor:

- If you have persistent **tingling** pins and needles or **numbness** in the fingers.
- If you have had an injury such as a **whiplash** following a car accident.
- If you have pain or swelling in the wrists or hands. (See **neuritis**.)

- If you have a **headache** accompanied by dizziness or nausea.
- If your headaches are becoming progressively worse.
- If your vision is becoming blurred.

NERVOUS SYSTEM

The central nervous system

This is the centre which directs and integrates all the functions of the human body. It consists of the brain, the complex computer system which sorts out all the nerve impulses, and the spinal cord. It provides the voluntary control of all activities and it is protected by the structures of the skull and the back. (See **anatomy**.)

The peripheral nervous system

This system, consisting of nerves, connects the central nervous system to all the areas of the body, and enables the brain to know what is happening everywhere in the body.

The nerves radiate out from the spinal cord. They vary in size from tiny microscopic threads to long fibres, such as the sciatic nerve which travels from your back to your toes. There are 31 pairs of spinal nerves and the branches come together from all over the body to enter the central column (the **spinal cord**) passing through the gaps in the **vertebrae**, the foramina.

There are two types of nerves forming the basic communication system between the central nervous system and the rest of the body. These are classified by their function:

Sensory nerves
To the rear of the spine, the sensory nerves enter the spinal cord through the posterior roots. These sensory nerves carry messages from the sense organs to the spinal cord and brain as a result of receiving external stimulation. Pain occurs when specific nerve endings are abnormally stimulated resulting in a motor nerve reaction.

Motor nerves
At the front of the spinal cord, the anterior nerve roots provide the motor pathways by which messages leave the spinal cord and are sent to the muscles of the body. If the back muscles receive the brain's messages of pain they try to protect the back by going into spasm.

The autonomic nervous system

This network of involuntary nerves, over which you have no conscious control, regulates the internal organs, such as the heart, lungs, liver, stomach, sex organs, bladder, kidneys and colon. The system is made up of two opposing networks, the sympathetic and parasympathetic, which connect with the spinal cord. It is strongly influenced by **emotions**, **stress** and **tension** in the human body. This system also travels in the spinal cord.

Nerve root compression
See **compression**.

NEURALGIA

This word comes from two Greek words, *neuron* nerve and *algos* pain. Neuralgia is thus an intense intermittent nerve pain, often felt in the arms and face. (See **brachialgia**.)

NEURITIS

This comes from the Greek words *neuron* meaning nerve, and *itis* meaning **inflammation**. This is inflammation of a nerve.

NEUROLOGY

The study of nerves – their anatomy and physiology.

NEUROLOGIST

The medical specialist who deals with the study and treatment of nerves. He is not involved in surgery.

NEUROSURGEON

A surgeon who operates on the **nervous system**.

NODULES

This is another description of the localised areas in muscle tissue which can be acutely painful on pressure. They are also described as **trigger points** or **knotted muscles**. (See **fibrositis**.)

NORSK SEQUENCE TRAINING MACHINES

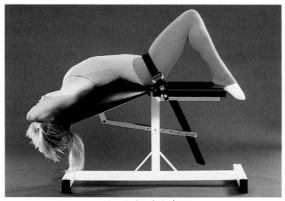

Norsk back trainer

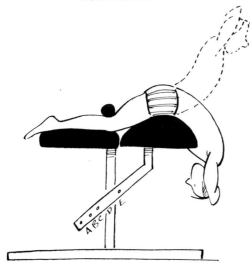

Norsk abdominal trainer

This equipment, designed and developed in Norway by two internationally known physiotherapists, Hans Gunnari and Olaf Evjenth, enables men and women, old and young, athletes or recuperating back patients, to improve muscular strength, endurance and mobility. (See gym equipment in Where to Get Help at the back of the book for details of distributors.)

NUCLEOUS PULPOSUS

See **disc**.

NUMBNESS

Prolonged pressure, or a more severe irritation, will result in the nerve supply being cut off. Numbness rather than pain in the nerve distribution of the back or legs can indicate a serious problem, so it is important to see a doctor. (See **compression**, **nervous system**.)

NURSES

Nurses play a large part in the hospitalisation of back patients, especially where bed rest, constant traction or severe injury is present. (See **hospital**.)

Bedmaking, **carrying** and **lifting** patients are all hazards for a nurse's back, but modern lifting and handling techniques have enabled the nursing profession to reduce back strain. Hoists, and an extremely useful **sling** developed by MeDesign, are available to overcome the problems of handling and lifting patients, saving undue stress on the back and reducing accidents and injuries.

NURSING MOTHERS

Posture and good support are extremely important when you are feeding a baby. Weak back muscles, **fatigue**, lack of sleep and poor furniture can all cause backache. (See **babies**.)

OBESITY

'Be fit, not fat!'

OBSERVATION

Start to look at other people's backs and their **posture** – in the street, at home, at the gym or while playing sport.

- Are they short or tall?
- Do they have a long back and long legs?
- Do they have a short back and long legs?
- Are they round shouldered?
- Do they carry their head on one side or poke out their chin?
- Do they have a stiff walk?
- Do they have a hollow back?

- Do they carry one shoulder higher than the other?
- Do they peer at the ground as they walk?
- How do they pick up their shopping in the supermarket?
- How do they carry suitcases or a school bag?
- How do they sit?

Learn to become observant, especially with your own family, and maybe you will be able to prevent back problems and help others to help themselves.

OFFICE

If you are stuck in an office all day, deskbound and perhaps unfit, there are several ways you can get into shape by doing **exercises** and purchasing the right **furniture.**

- Check your sitting **posture** frequently.
- Practise **neck** exercises.

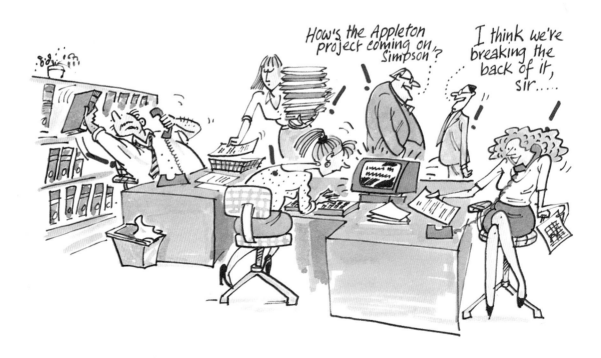

- Do *extension* exercises, leaning on the desk to press up and stretch.
- Do squats, holding on to the back of the chair. (See *squatting*.)
- Get up at regular intervals and walk round the office. (See *walking*.)
- Go out in your lunch hour and buy furniture that is ergonomically suitable for your back. (See *ergonomics*.)

ORGANISATIONS

There are many organisations which you can contact, either for help with back problems or for specialist treatment. (See the Where To Get Help section at the end of the book.)

ORTHOPAEDICALLY DESIGNED

This is a 'buzz' word from the 1960s.

ORTHOPAEDICS

This is the branch of medicine which relates to *bones*, *joints*, *muscles* and related structures. If surgery is necessary for your back it may be performed by an orthopaedic surgeon, who is also trained to manipulate under anaesthetic when more conservative manipulative procedures have failed. (See *manipulation*.) *Nurses* and chartered *physiotherapists* may also train specifically in orthopaedic medicine.

ORTHOTISTS

Orthotists are responsible for providing *braces* and splinting that may be required for the back, for example a plaster of Paris jacket, a brace or a *corset*. They work in close cooperation with the surgeon and doctor.

OSTEOARTHRITIS

See *osteoarthrosis*.

OSTEOARTHROSIS

This is one of the names that is given to the process of degenerative *arthritis*. (See *degeneration*.) Degenerative arthritis is correctly called osteoarthrosis and it has nothing to do with rheumatoid arthritis. Everyone after the age of 21 experiences some degree of osteoarthrosis according to their lifestyle and activities – degeneration occurs in the *discs* and *facet joints*, where a certain degree of wear and tear is inevitable.

When you are young, the repair processes of the body keep up with any wear and tear, but as you get older the body gets slower in healing, muscles become weaker, cartilage is lost and the lubricated joint surfaces become rougher and grate together.

Pain may result in the back as a result of:

- A lack of shock absorption.
- Protective muscle *spasm*.
- The formation of new bone which appears at the edges of ageing joints as 'spurs' of bone. (See *osteophyte*.)

Osteoarthrosis is often detected early in younger people who do regular excessive exercise programmes for activities such as gymnastics and athletics. It is therefore important to have growing children checked regularly.

What to do

- Keep moving as 'man is made to move'.
- Have *heat therapy* to improve local *circulation*.
- Wear *supports* to help painful joints. (See *collar*, *corset*.)
- Maintain good *posture* constantly.
- Perform gentle light *exercise* on a regular basis.
- Buy the correct *furniture*.

- Drive the right **car** for your back.
- Maintain an activity such as **walking**, **cycling** or **swimming**.

You should seek professional medical advice if you are worried about this condition, but remember it happens to all of us.

OSTEOCHONDRITIS

The cause of osteochondritis is unknown. It is an **inflammation** in part of a **joint** which causes pain and deformity, mainly affecting the **cartilage**. It usually occurs in adolescence. (See **Scheuermann's disease**.)

OSTEOPATHY

This system of healing was founded in 1874 by Doctor Andrew Taylor Still in Missouri, USA, and was originally based on the idea that all disease resulted from spinal derangements. Osteopathy is a physical manipulative therapy. It is mainly concerned with the **diagnosis** and treatment of musculoskeletal disorders to restore full mobility to any spinal **joint** in which the osteopath considers there is restricted movement. **Manipulation** is not performed if disease is present. Practitioners also believe that spinal problems influence the nervous control of other organs such as the lungs or stomach, so osteopathy is not limited to movement alone.

Osteopath

When you see an osteopath, a full history of your back is taken and the back is examined by using detailed **palpation** and by moving the **joints** through their full range to see where there is restricted movement, which may be responsible for the problems elsewhere. Osteopaths employ different articulatory techniques according to the needs of the individual patient. Massage-like release movements to relax muscles and soft tissues, passive repetitive joint movements and high velocity thrust techniques are performed

which sometimes produce a 'click'.

A registered osteopath will have trained for four years but if you are in doubt about consulting one, ask your doctor's advice first. The letters MRO will identify a registered osteopath.

OSTEOPHYTES

These bony outgrowths appear at the edges of ageing **joints**; they develop over a long period as part of the process of growing old. The size and position of an osteophyte can sometimes interfere with other structures, and this can cause pain, but more often they do not interfere with the functions of the back. (See **bones, degeneration, osteoarthrosis, compression**.)

OSTEOPOROSIS

Osteoporosis literally means porous bones. It has been considered a natural phenomena with ageing, but it is a medical problem that affects older people. It has been found that osteoporosis is alarmingly common; although it affects both men and women, it is most likely to occur in women after the **menopause** – about 3 million women in the UK past the age of menopause suffer from it.

Research has found that the mineral metabolism associated with ageing of the musculoskeletal system is responsible. In the back it occurs in the **vertebrae**, where the bones become thin, weak and more fragile, producing increased stooping or 'dowager's hump', and the vertebrae may even collapse or fracture under stress. (See **kyphosis, posture**.) The back will become weaker still and more fragile unless an activity such as **walking** and a short programme of **exercises** is performed two or three times a week.

Diet, **vitamins**, hormone replacement therapy and retaining an active life by doing regular exercise are all essential in order to limit osteoporosis, and investigations and research are currently underway to find further help for this condition.

OVERWEIGHT

'Great eaters and great sleepers are incapable of anything else that is great.'
King Henry IV France, 1553-1610

If you are overweight, you may eventually feel it in your back. All the weight-carrying joints will suffer as they cannot support the stress caused by abnormal loads, which can increase the rate of **degeneration** in the joints. The lumbar curve of the spine increases and backache and strain may result. The **abdominal muscles** become stretched and weak, and the back muscles have to work overtime as a result. (See **bio-mechanics**, **lordosis**.) The strain of carrying extra weight can also affect the heart and blood vessels.

'Be fit not fat.'

OVERWORK

'No work is worse than overwork.'
Charles Lamb, 1775-1834

PAGET'S DISEASE

A rare **bone** disease which occurs in the ageing back, resulting in an irregular thickening of the outer layer of bone. An **X-ray** will show the irregular bone density in the back, but Paget's disease is not confined to the vertebrae. It may start with pain in the hips, legs or arms, although it is more often associated with the back.

PAIN

'For all the happiness mankind can gain,
Is not in pleasure but in rest from pain.'

Cortez

Pain is a symptom of many back conditions and it is most commonly felt in the **lumbar region**. It is only a sign that something is wrong, but it can be a frightening experience. It may be:

- A sharp, intense, sudden jabbing pain.
- A constant, dull persistent pain.
- A discomfort.
- A mild ache.

Don't just hope that it will go away; it will probably become worse. You will probably be very aware of it, so try and identify your pain, then find out the cause immediately and do something about it, otherwise pain leads to fear, fear leads to **tension**, and tension leads to more pain, so you are in a vicious circle. This circle must be broken if you are to have relief from pain. (See **acute back**, **help**, **positions**.)

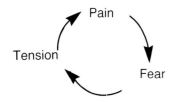

Some causes of back pain

- Mechanical injuries causing joint **inflammation**. (See **biomechanics**, **joints**, **sprain**, **strain**.)
- Lack of movement leading to **stiffness**.
- Muscle **spasm**.
- A **disc** prolapse, bony outgrowths, or pressure on nerves, **ligaments** or the **spinal cord**. (See **compression**, **osteophytes**.)
- **Fractures**.
- Pinched **fat**. (See **fascia**.)
- **Ankylosing spondylitis**.
- Gynaecological problems.
- Indigestion.

If you have pain for over 24 hours, see your doctor.

Referred pain

Pain originating in one part of the body but felt at another site after being transmitted through the network of nerves is known as referred pain.

For example, you can often feel pain down the leg when really the root of the pain is coming from a disturbance of the nerves in the back. (See **compression**.) The area of the leg and the region of the back share the same nerve supply and the brain misinterprets the real source of the pain. (See **sciatica**.)

A thorough examination and tests by a qualified medical practitioner usually determine the site of referred pain.

Exercises which may help pain

Depending on the cause of the back pain, the shape of your lower back, the site of the problem and whether it is acute or chronic, you can do these **exercises** both in a passive and active way to help relieve the pain and prevent further episodes. It is very important that you observe any changes in the area of your pain and notice whether the pain gets worse or better. Be cautious and do not hurry.

If the pain makes you bend forwards
Lie flat, face down on a firm surface, with a pillow under the tummy. Slowly withdraw the pillow from under the tummy as the pain subsides, until you can lie flat with a pillow supporting the head and neck only. Gravity flattens you out in this passive exercise until gradually you can place more pillows under the chest to ease the lower back into a natural curve.

If the pain is alleviated by this exercise, you can progress to further **extension exercises**.

If the pain is felt from bending forwards
Stand upright with your feet slightly apart at shoulder width. Place your hands in the small of your back and bend the trunk backwards as far as you can, keeping the knees straight. Hold for one or two counts. Return to the starting position. Repeat five times.
NOTE: It is important to correct your **posture** for back comfort at this stage.

If the pain makes you extend the lower back
In this situation the **facet joints** are **jammed**, subsequently pinching the tissues. (See **lordosis**.) The **flexion position** is very useful if you have **acute back** pain and the surrounding muscles are tight and aching.

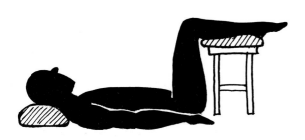

Lying flat on your back, with the head and neck well supported on pillows, bend the knees and hips to a full angle of 90 degrees and support them on a small stool or pillows in order to relax the small muscles at the front of the hip joints and all the painful structures in the back. When the pain is less acute, you can progress to **pelvic tilt** and further **flexion** and **mobilising exercises**.
NOTE: It is important to check your **posture** at this stage. Remember, poor posture hurts.

PAIN KILLERS

A wide range of **drugs** for the relief of back pain is available to doctors for prescription and over the counter at the local chemist. Simple painkillers, such as **aspirin** and paracetamol, and other more powerful products will all help alleviate back pain, by:

- Relaxing **muscles**.
- Acting as an **analgesic**.
- Relieving **inflammation**.

NOTE: Use the time when you have relief from pain to discover the cause of the pain.

PAIN MANAGEMENT CLINICS

These clinics are part of most **hospital** services. They have a non-surgical approach to pain, using one or a number of the following techniques:

- Neurostimulation with a **transcutaneous nerve stimulator**.
- **Relaxation** techniques.
- **Hypnotherapy**.
- **Drug** therapy, where it is necessary.

PALPATION

The application of the fingers to feel and assess tone and sensitivity in the joints and muscles of the back is known as palpation. It enables the practitioner to discover tenderness, **spasm** and **pain**, and it accustoms you to the feel of the hands for further manual therapy. (See **acupressure**, **Maitland**, **manipulation**, **massage**.)

PARACHUTING

This, together with sky diving, is probably one of the worst activities for the back and can cause horrific accidents.

PARASTHESIA

Parasthesia is the medical term describing the peculiar feelings of **tingling**, **pins and needles**, burning or prickling caused by **compression** on a nerve. (See **disc** bulge.)

PARTNERS

See **beds**.

PELVIS

The pelvis is a strong bony arch, articulating above with the **lumbar region** and below with the thigh bones. (See **anatomy**.) It consists of three bones:

- The triangular-shaped **sacrum** sandwiched between the two **ilia**.
- The sacrum joins the ilia at the **sacroiliac joints**.
- The ilia are attached in front where the pubic bones come together at the symphysis pubis.

What the pelvis does

- It provides the foundation for the backbones to rest on.
- Its most important function is to transfer body weight from the back to the legs by acting as a large hinge. It joins the head and the trunk to the legs by way of two sockets in the ilia which, with the heads of the thigh bones, form the hip joints.
- It encircles, supports and protects certain internal organs – the bladder, the colon, the rectum and, in women, the uterus. The pelvis of the female is wider and shallower than that of a male.

PELVIC TILT

The position of the **pelvis** controls the **balance** of the back and the body. The pelvic tilt is therefore the most important thing to learn for strong stable good **posture** and to avoid mechanical strain for activities such as **lifting**.
NOTE: Practise the pelvic tilt every day, like cleaning your teeth.

Lying

Lie on your back on the floor or a firm bed with your knees bent and slightly apart, your feet on the floor. The head and neck should be supported with a pillow and your arms should be by your sides. The hips and knees should be at a comfortable angle, about 45 degrees.

Place the back of one hand between the floor and the hollow of your back. Press down, flatten your waist and lower the back firmly and gently on to your hand by tightening your **abdominal muscles** and squeezing your buttocks. Don't arch the back or hold your breath. Hold for five counts and relax for five. Feel the pelvis tilting up and back – think about it – and then feel it roll out of position as you relax.

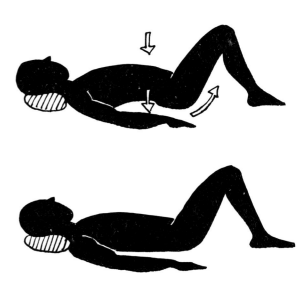

NOTE: It is important to think about what you are doing, what it feels like and how to control it, so it becomes a good habit.

Sitting

Sit on a firm chair with good support, head erect with the chin pulled in, the shoulders relaxed and the arms by your sides.

Tighten and pull in your tummy muscles, so again the pelvis is tilted up and forwards and the buttocks are clenched. Hold for five and relax. Repeat slowly five to ten times.

Standing

Stand with your back against a wall to help you feel the position. Keep the head erect with the chin pulled in and the shoulders relaxed. Breathe normally.

Pull in your tummy muscles and tighten your buttocks, feeling the pelvis tilting upwards and forwards at the symphysis pubis. Hold for five and relax. Repeat five to ten times until you really know the movement.

PERIODS

Backache is often present in the lower back before a monthly period. Most women retain fluids at this time, which puts extra pressure on the tissues and subsequently the **joints**, making you feel uncomfortable and bloated, with a dragging dull ache in the back. **Abdominal muscle** tone can become poor.

It is important to keep active and make sure that no internal interference is occurring due to tampons, a diaphragm, or an intrauterine device. Warmth, a **painkiller** and perhaps a diuretic to cut down on the fluid retention, prescribed by the doctor, can help. Seek medical advice to make sure it is nothing serious. (See **acute back**, **gynaecology**, **heat therapy**.)

PERIPHERAL NERVES

These are the nerves radiating out from the back and descending into the arms and legs, relaying sensations, working **muscles**, and transmitting pain from the back. (See **nervous system**.)

PHYSIOLOGY

The science of the functions of the body.

PHYSIOTHERAPY

Physiotherapy can play a vital part in pain relief, healing and rehabilitation of the back. Physiotherapy incorporates a wide range of skills including **massage**, **manipulation**, **mobilisation**, and **exercises**, often aided by sophisticated electronic and electrical apparatus or acupuncture.

Preventative medicine is a very important aspect of physiotherapy. During treatment, time is spent looking at the causes of the pain, teaching the patient how to avoid a recurrence of the back problem by postural correction, re-education and **relaxation** techniques for stress related problems. (See Appendix for the address of the Chartered Society of Physiotherapy.)

'If it is physical it is therapy.'

Physiotherapist

This profession is recognised by the letters MCSP, member of the Chartered Society of Physiotherapy, in the UK. All physiotherapists have a minimum of three years training.

Physiotherapists can treat back pain using a wide range of techniques including:

- **Massage**.
- **Mobilisations**.
- **Manipulation**.
- **Exercises**.
- **Acupuncture**.
- **Electrotherapy**.

The chartered physiotherapist will look at the causes of the pain and help the patient learn how to avoid its recurrence in the future. A programme of exercises and postural re-education will be given to guarantee a high standard of treatment.

PIANO PLAYING

A round curved back and shoulders can result from piano playing if the stool is not at the correct level for the keys. (See **kyphosis**.) It is therefore important that the stool should be adjustable, especially for a growing child, and the music should be correctly placed to prevent the head poking forwards with a subsequent neckache. (See **chairs**, **neck**, **posture**.)

PILLOWS

Pillows are for comfort and **support**. A good pillow or pillows are essential for positioning the back correctly, especially when lying, sleeping and sitting. Support for the head and neck, and for the natural **curves** of the spine, both when lying on the back and on the side, will prevent discomfort and avoid back strain. (See **beds**, **positions**, **posture**, **Pro-Pil-o**, **Sommelier**.)

- If you sleep on your back, place a pillow under your knees.
- If you sleep on your side, place a pillow between your knees and ankles.
- If you sleep on too many pillows, the **neck** will be stretched and straight, resulting in **morning stiffness**.

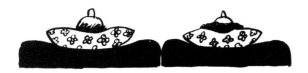

PINS AND NEEDLES

This expression describes the feeling of sharp **tingling** which arises when there is pressure on a nerve. (See **compression**.)

PLASTER OF PARIS

Plaster of Paris is used to make a brace or jacket for immobilisation after surgery to the back, following a severe injury or a fracture. They can be heavy and uncomfortable, especially in hot weather, but they are excellent for protection and rehabilitation.

A plentiful supply of talcum powder will prevent too much irritation under the plaster, while a good oil massage for the skin when the plaster is removed will feel marvellous.

PODIATRIST

A podiatrist, DPM, is trained to treat structural problems of the **feet** as well as other common foot complaints that are usually treated by a **chiropodist**. A podiatrist can be extremely helpful with advice on feet and **shoes**, which in turn will be of help for the back when **walking** and **running**.

POSITIONS

Positions and positioning are very important in back care. Correct positioning is the easiest way to help your back pain, especially in the acute stage. (See **acute back**.) If you have back pain, it is often difficult to get from lying down to sitting and standing positions. Resuming the erect **posture** should be performed correctly, otherwise more undue stress and strain will be placed on the back. **Pillows** can be extremely helpful for positioning the back in lying down when there is acute pain, or when sitting, to maintain the natural curves of the back.

Be aware of the following activities and the

positions you use in them every day; adapt them if necessary, to make sure you are helping your back:

- **Resting** in the lying position.
- Sitting in a **chair** with good **support**.
- **Standing**, with a good **posture**.
- **Carrying** things.
- **Lifting** things.
- **Exercise**, using the arms and legs.
- **Breathing** and **relaxation**.
- **Foot** movements.
- **Sex**.
- **Sport**.

Lying down

This is the most comfortable position and posture for the back if you have **pain**, providing you are on a firm supportive surface. (See **beds**.) The spine elongates during sleep after the effort of standing all day. The natural **curves** of the back, which have become exaggerated, flatten out when you lie down, and the **discs** are able to absorb fluid in minute quantities.

If there is severe muscle **spasm** or advanced **arthritis**, then lying still for too long can aggravate the back, so **mobilising movements** or frequent rolling from side to side will help. Lying on the stomach can increase back problems if they are caused by exaggerated **extension** of the back.

The foetal position exercise

A very comfortable position when there is low back pain is the foetal position. It is possible to exercise gently in bed in this position, to start mobilising the back.

Lie on your side, keeping the legs and knees together with the knees slightly bent up. Slowly and gently curl up, pulling the knees towards each other in a primary C curve. Hold for a count of five, then gently uncurl.
NOTE: If you have any pain with this exercise, don't do it.

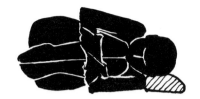

Foetal position

POSTNATAL

Postnatal exercises will help counteract tiredness and strengthen muscles which may have become stretched and weakened during **pregnancy**. They will also prevent further problems arising in later years. (See **pelvic tilt**, **posture** and Suggested Further Reading.)

POSTURE

'What's a fine person or a beauteous face,
Unless deportment gives them decent grace.'
Winston Churchill, 1874-1965

The dictionary states that 'posture is the relative position of the body in space, the position of the body in relation to itself and the surrounding environment'. Posture is both static and dynamic, and in order to take care of your back you should be aware and understand the importance of posture.

- Static posture is when you are lying, sitting or standing still.
- Dynamic or active posture is the changing posture of the body when **carrying**, **lifting**, **walking** and all the other activities of daily living.

For good posture, the natural **curves** of the back are in balance with one another, allowing the back to work with the *minimum of effort and the minimum of stress*.

Military posture

People who stand with their shoulders braced back, the feet turned out and an exaggerated low back curve, such as is seen in a military posture, will get back pain from this stance. Excessive *lordosis*, a thrust out 'pigeon' chest and stiff rigid shoulders, as well as carrying heavy equipment, will lead to back problems.

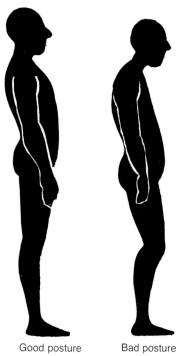

Good posture   Bad posture

Standing

Avoid *standing* with slouched shoulders, a rounded back or a protruding abdomen, as this places constant stress on the *ligaments*, *muscles* and *joints* of the back.

Always try to stand in a balanced position with your weight on both feet, not on one leg like a stork or a ballet dancer. The shoulders should be relaxed, with the neck and the chin tucked in. Place a fingertip on the crown of your head; then try and think tall, reaching upwards with the crown of your head.

Sitting

Sitting places greater stress on the lower back than standing does. It is important to maintain the natural curves of the back while you are sitting down. (See *chairs, Mandal, office, supports, workplace*.)

Lying

Since you spend about one-third of your life in *bed*, it is important that good static posture is maintained in this position. (See *pillows, positions*.)

The posture checklist

Much of the stress of daily living can be reduced by careful planning of where and how you work. Check these points:

- Position for *sleeping*. Do I have enough *pillows* for support? Do I have too many pillows? Is my mattress firm or sagging?
- Posture getting in and out of *bed*? Do I know how?
- Posture for cleaning teeth and shaving. Are the basin and mirror at the right height?
- Posture for turning on the bath taps? Am I *bending* correctly?
- Posture for making the bed? Do I need fitted sheets and a duvet?
- Loading the dishwasher. Am I doing it correctly?
- Getting in and out of the *car*? Am I *twisting* my back?
- Is my posture correct at *work*? Am I sitting for too long? Is the telephone in the correct position? Is the height of the desk and VDU correct?
- Do I know the correct position for vacuuming and other *housework*?
- How should I mow the lawn and weed the flowerbeds when *gardening*?
- Do I know how to stand correctly at a cocktail party or wedding reception?
- Do I know the correct posture for watching television?

How many negative answers have you? Go back and read the relevant sections again.

It may take weeks or months to re-educate your posture so that you have a natural *balance* and poise. A back school organised by a chartered *physiotherapist*, *Alexander Technique* or *Feldenkrais* teacher can help you.

'Practice makes perfect.'

PREGNANCY

It is wise to take extra care of your back during the nine months of pregnancy; statistics show that nine out of ten women suffer with back pain at some time in this period.

- A hormone is produced during pregnancy which softens and stretches the **sacroiliac ligaments** to allow an easy passage of the baby through the **pelvis.**
- The added weight of the baby in front causes postural alterations. You have to alter your **balance** and put your centre of gravity further back towards the heels than you did before pregnancy, causing subsequent **strain** to the facet **joints** of the back, especially in the lower back and on the sacroiliac joints. (See **biomechanics**, **posture**, **sacrum**.)
- The excessive **lordosis**, which may be caused by weak **abdominal muscles** of the pregnant mother, with the tummy pushed forwards and the bottom backwards creating a hollow back, results in poor posture. If all the antigravity **muscles** are strong and the **ligaments** have not become too relaxed, you will avoid back-ache. (See **pelvic tilt**.)
- Wearing high heels during pregnancy upsets balance, causing instability and pain in the back. (See **feet, shoes**.)

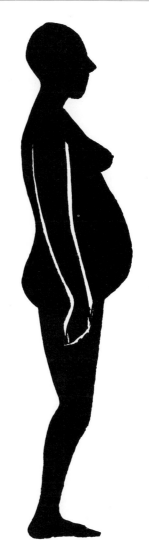

Posture during pregnancy

Useful tips

It can take five to six months for the ligaments to tighten up after childbirth, so it is important to take the following precautions to avoid weak overstretched ligaments and muscles, which will in turn cause back strain.

- Practise good posture every day in front of a **mirror**.
- Learn how to correct your **pelvic tilt**.
- Avoid wearing high heels or shoes with a small base such as a stiletto, which will only throw your weight further forwards. Flat or wide medium heels are best.

- Take care **lifting** and **carrying** children, especially if it is a second or subsequent pregnancy, and avoid lifting heavy weights. (See **babies**.)
- Try and get help manoeuvring furniture, or when **pushing** a pram or shopping. Put parcels in a trolley, in a shopping basket on wheels, or arrange for someone to carry them for you.
- Have your ironing board high enough so you do not have to stoop. Or lower the board and sit down on a chair or stool. (See **housework**.)

- If there is weakness in the muscles or acute pain in the back, ask if you can wear a pregnancy **corset** or belt. This can either have an expandable elastic front or it can be a wide webbing belt worn round the sacroiliac joints and underneath the bulge to give good support.
- Rest and **relaxation** should be frequent and enjoyable.
- Attend **antenatal** and **postnatal** classes to learn exercises and to prepare for birth and motherhood. (See **childbirth**, **exercises**, **positions**, **squatting**, Where to Get Help and Suggested Further Reading.)

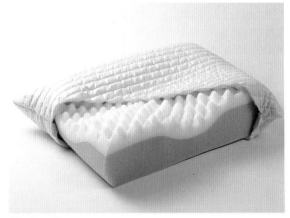

The Pro-Pil-o

PRESSURE

See **compression**.

PREVENTION

'An ounce of prevention – a pound of cure.'

PRO-PIL-O

Because one of the most common causes of **neck** and **shoulder** pain is incorrect **posture** during sleep, the use of a Pro-Pil-o for support and correct head and neck alignment will help you to sleep. The **pillow** offers support for the **cervical region** of the spine in its natural curves and provides even support of the neck in sleeping on the side. It is designed to cradle the head and protect the neck by a choice of two different comfort levels, using convoluted foam like an egg crate which spreads the weight and allows the circulation of air. The Pro-Pil-o also has a non-allergic cover.

PSYCHOLOGICAL BACK PROBLEMS

A psychological back is usually caused by **emotions** or **stress**; pain is perceived that has no discernible organic cause. A human behavioural psychologist, a good physician or a qualified counsellor will be of help to establish if you are a tense or very highly strung person with:

- Emotional problems.
- Problems at work.
- Financial problems.
- Marital problems.

A stress-related back disorder is now recognised as a medical condition, and after you have been assessed carefully you can be taught to cope with these problems.

PUBS

A high bar stool can be a hazard in a pub, especially if it has no supporting rungs for the feet and your legs are left dangling in mid-air. It is better to lean squarely on the bar and stretch the back gently, or stand with one foot on the footrail rather than sitting on a stool and propping yourself up on one elbow. (See **posture**, **sitting**.)

PUSHING AND PULLING

Both these actions are hazardous for the back unless performed correctly and with thought. Foot stability and body weight are the main factors governing the strength of pushing and pulling, with the strength of the *legs* and *shoulder* muscles also playing a significant part. (See *biomechanics*, *feet*, *positions*.)

Pushing

Stresses on the back are usually higher for pushing than pulling. The shoulders have to push the load and the ribcage stiffens, which can make *breathing* difficult. The *abdominal muscles* and back muscles work to move the object, and the application of the horizontal forces involved in the push can cause the feet to slip.

If you have to push a car or heavy object, lean

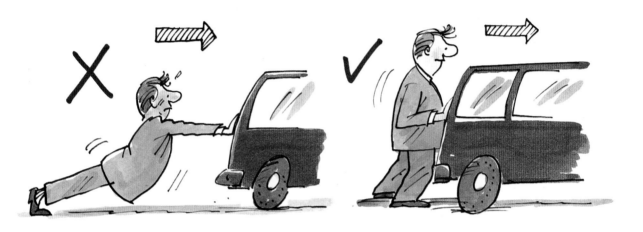

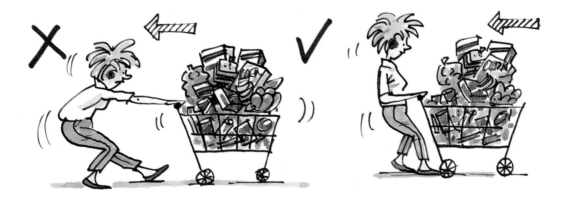

the back on the object to be moved, and use the thigh and leg muscles to minimise the stress on the back. The back is kept erect and you can breathe freely and use your abdominal muscle with correct **pelvic tilt**.

Rules for pushing

- Pushing the car, or any other heavy object, should be performed carefully, observing the rules for **lifting**.
- The strength of the push required will depend mainly on foot stability and on body weight.
- Use your arms and legs, and tighten the abdominal muscles when pushing.
- Keep your arms bent for pushing.
- Make sure you have good wheels on a trolley or pram.
- When you have finished pushing an object check your pelvic tilt and **posture**.

Pulling

When you pull, you need to **twist** and exert pressure on the spine, causing undue forces on the back and neck. However, in a straight pull, the force can be applied fairly close to the backbone, near the body, with the feet placed firmly on the ground. (See **levers**.)

Rules for pulling

- Remember to take the strain on your leg and arm muscles rather than your back.
- Keep the object you are pulling close to the body and hold it firmly.
- Stand with your feet apart, bend your knees and crouch slightly to pull the object. (See **bending**.)
- Lean away from the object and pull it by straightening your legs, keeping the back straight.

- Move backwards slowly and carefully, with the knees slightly bent so the legs take the strain.
- When you have finished pulling, check your pelvic tilt and posture.

PUTNAM

James Putnam designed the first orthopaedic drivers' seat for London taxis in the 1970s. Today about three-quarters of black-cab owner-drivers

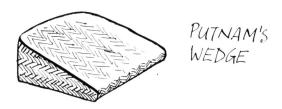

PUTNAM'S
WEDGE

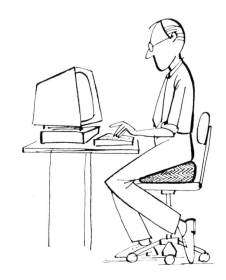

in London use Putnam's Flyer car seat. Another product, a very comfortable lumbar **support** cushion, the Putnam's Backrest, is available in two sizes, and James Putnam has also developed other back care products which are recommended by medical practitioners, such as, the sitting **wedge**, which adapts an ordinary office **chair** by changing the seat angle 10 degrees, and inflatable lumbar rolls and travel **pillows** for adults and children. (See **cars**.)

QUADRICEPS

These four *muscles* at the front of the thigh have to be strong to help the back in *lifting, pushing* and many other movements. They should be in good *tone* for a good *posture*. (See *knees*.)

QUESTIONS

If in doubt, ask a question.

Here are some questions that you should ask yourself before you go rushing to the doctor.

- Is your back fit enough to handle your work without discomfort or pain? (See *ergonomics, housework, workplace*.)
- Is the *furniture* and other equipment at work and at home adequately designed for your back? (See *beds, chairs*.)
- Is your mattress over ten years old?
- Have you been *lifting* too much shopping, heavy furniture or luggage recently?
- Does another member of your family have a history of back problems? (See *congenital*.)
- Have you suddenly started wearing high-heeled *shoes*?
- If you are a child have you suddenly grown?
- Are you bothered physically by *backache*, constipation, muscle *spasm*, or a *headache*?
- Have you had a recent *coughing* or *sneezing* fit?
- Have you had a *holiday* this year?
- Have you started a programme of *exercise*?
- Can you turn your head to look over each shoulder? (See *neck*.)
- Have you twisted suddenly to look at someone? (See *twisting*.)
- Have you been for a walk lately? (See *walking*.)

- Do you sit for a long time in front of the television in a sagging slumped *posture*?
- Are you depressed? (See *depression*.)
- Are you overworked and run down? (See *stress*.)
- Are you getting in the car to do everything? (See *exercise*.)
- Have you been very athletic, but stopped for a long period without any *activity* because of the pressure of work? (See *exercise, stress*.)
- Have you backache because you've stopped work and become bored and depressed because you feel you are missing something? (See *psychological back problems*.)

Ask yourself some of these questions, and with the use of this book you may find the cause of your back problem before seeking out the doctor's advice. If you are in doubt, see the doctor.

Questions the doctor may ask

- When was the first time you had any back trouble?
- Have you changed your style of living lately?
- Have you had back *pain* before? How many times? When? Was it as bad as now?
- Is there any back trouble in your family? (See *congenital*.)
- What other physical signs have you? (See *examination*.)
- Have you been under any *stress* recently?
- Do you have a heavy manual job, or is it sedentary? (See *lifting, office*.)
- Did the pain start gradually or suddenly?
- What helps the pain? What makes it worse?
- Have you ever had a fall or been injured – a car accident, a fall from a horse, or skiing?
- Did you have a normal *pregnancy* and *childbirth*?
- Do *coughing, sneezing* or bladder and bowel movements affect your back?

This history of your back condition will help the doctor, although a lot of the questions are similar to the ones you can ask yourself.

RACK

This expression is often used for **traction** treatment, which has been a remedy for back problems since ancient times.

READING

A relaxed position for the arms, **neck** and head, and a well-supported back, are all essential to avoid back and neck **strain** while holding and reading a book or newspaper. (See **chairs**, **supports**.) Poor eyesight may cause back problems; if you find you are peering at the paper with your head poking forwards, maybe your **eyes** need testing or you are ready for new spectacles. (See **copyholder**.) Reading in **bed** may seem like a good idea, but unless **pillows** are really giving proper support you will have a **crick** in the neck and aching arms, which will lead to disturbed sleep and **morning stiffness** the next day.

REBOUNDING

The design of rebounders evolved from trampolining, which was invented by George Nissen of America in 1936. Recent research on the subject was published in 1977 by Albert Carter, based on Sir Isaac Newton's laws of gravity.

Rebounding is a convenient and enjoyable way of taking **aerobic** exercise. It is safer for a back that has suffered from the impact of **jarring** or shock on the spine during **running**, **jogging** or playing tennis. It is not a good exercise for chronic joint problems of the back. (See **chronic back**, **joints**, **sport**.)

REFERRED PAIN

See **pain**.

REFLEXOLOGY

Reflexology, which originated in ancient Egypt, is the use of the hands to massage particular areas of the hands and feet, where certain points reflect each organ of the body. It employs many **acupuncture** and **shiatsu** principles and is specific to each individual. The effects of the treatment are relayed to the whole body by a flow and balance of energy through the **meridians**. It can help a painful back and headaches unless acute circulatory problems or infections and disease are present. The International School of Reflex Zone Therapy began in Germany in 1956 and reflexology is now widely used all over the world. (See Where to Get Help.)

REGISTERED

It is important to check that the medical practitioner who is treating your back has the proper qualifications and is registered with the relevant authority.

RELAXATION

It is vitally important to have plenty of relaxation. Relaxation takes away all the **stresses** that you place upon yourself and your back in everyday life, so it is important to examine your lifestyle and make time for relaxation.

The art of relaxation will only come with practice. Try for ten minutes every day, preferably lying down to take the weight off your back and feet. Let go and let the mind think of something really nice, or just let it go blank. Make sure the eyelids are relaxed, and you may find you are asleep.

Letting go

Relaxation should be practised in a warm room. Remove your shoes, and loosen tight clothing. A restful atmosphere should be created, so lighting should be dim, and soft music may be helpful.

Lie on your back on a firm **bed** or on the floor, with a **pillow** under the head and your arms by your sides or resting on your tummy. Place a pillow under the knees. If you prefer to sleep on your front, or side, you may find it more comfortable to relax this way, with one arm raised and one leg bent. (See **positions**, **supports**.)

Let go, starting with the feet first. Tighten up the **muscles** of the feet and then let them go. Gradually work upwards with the calves, thighs, buttocks, stomach, chest, arms, hands, shoulders and neck. Finally screw up the face and then let go, with the eyes shut and the whole body feeling floppy and droopy.

Listen to your breathing. (See **breathing exercises**.) It should be deep and regular. Let your mind go blank, think lovely thoughts, or listen to music.

NOTE: If you are not able to lie down for complete relaxation, practise when sitting or standing, even if it is just facial relaxation and closing your eyes for a few minutes. Gentle stroking **massage** and attending **yoga** classes may also help you achieve general relaxation.

REPETITIVE MOVEMENTS

Vague aches and pains in the back usually arise from repetitive movements during **housework**, typing and other forms of manual work. This repetition **strains** the same structures every day and it is necessary to break the pattern to prevent more serious **chronic back** problems. (See **ergonomics**, **office**, **workplace**.) Think about the way you do various tasks and see if there are alternative actions to avoid repetitive strain.

RESPIRATION

See **breathing exercises**.

RESEARCH

Continual research is going on into the causes of back pain, how to prevent it and what treatments are really valid. The National Back Pain Association is the charity which raises money to further these objectives and provide help for sufferers. (See Where To Get Help section at the end of the book.)

REST

Absolute **bed** rest is necessary in the case of an **acute back** condition. It is one of the most important parts of the treatment and can sometimes prevent further problems. It is important to:

- Always rest on a firm supportive mattress.
- Use a bed board under the mattress if the bed is too soft.
- Don't lie flat on your back for too long without moving as it will cause **stiffness**, wasting **muscles** and subsequent weakness.

    Avoid inactivity as most back conditions are due to lack of mobility in one or more **joints**. Early mobilisation with adequate rest is the answer. (See **mobilising exercises**.) If a back joint is acutely inflamed and the **disc** and nerve have a lot of pressure, then bed rest is the ideal answer, but fidgeting and moving around in the bed will prevent total immobilisation – even getting on and off a bedpan provides activity. (See **positions**, **hospital**.)

'Too much rest can cause rust.'

RHEUMATISM

An expression often used by the general public to describe a whole range of **backaches**, diseases, pains and symptoms involving bones, joints and muscles. It should not be confused with *rheumatoid arthritis*, and is just a general term.

RHEUMATOID ARTHRITIS

Rheumatoid **arthritis** is a painful and disabling disease, the **diagnosis** of which is confirmed by **X-rays** and other laboratory tests. It should not be confused with **osteoarthritis**.

Rheumatoid arthritis often starts in middle life by changes taking place in the **joints**, causing general stiffness, deformity and restriction of movement. The joints in the limbs become inflamed and red, but those in the back may often not be affected until later. (See **inflammation**.) Rheumatoid arthritis can attack the top two **vertebrae**, the **atlas** and the **axis**, damaging and weakening the **ligaments** that tie them together and bind the vertebrae to the skull. This, together with the swelling in the joints, compresses the **spinal cord** and the lower part of the skull.

If you think you have rheumatoid arthritis, seek medical advice and help immediately from a **doctor** and a **rheumatologist**.

RHEUMATOLOGIST

This is the specialist dealing with **rheumatoid arthritis**, **osteoarthrosis** and other forms of **arthritis**. (See **ankylosing spondylitis**.) Treatment will include **anti-inflammatory** drugs, **injections** and **physiotherapy**.

RIBS

Twelve pairs of ribs attach to the spine in the **thoracic region**, the middle back. They form a cage which is attached to the breastbone, the sternum, at the front of the chest. This cage protects the heart and lungs.

The ribs move every time you take a breath, lifting upwards and outwards as the lungs expand to fill with air. They expel stale air as you breath out, when the ribs move down and in. (See **breathing exercises**.)

If the tissues surrounding the ribs become inflamed during a bout of **bronchitis** or pleurisy, it can cause pain in the back. (See **inflammation**.)

RICKED BACK

An expression used to explain a wrench or tear of **ligaments** or **muscles**, with a probable **locking** of the **joints** in the back.

RIDING

Horse riding is an enjoyable activity, but if you have had a fall, an injury or back problems where **ligaments** have become overstretched, such as after **pregnancy** and **childbirth**, riding may cause further **backache** and pain, because of the continuous **vibration** on the back due to movements such as trotting and forward **bending** when jumping. (See **coccydinia**, **repetitive movements**.)

ROCKING

This is an excellent movement for the back to mobilise the **lumbar region**. (See **mobilising exercises**.) A rocking **chair** provides continual motion for the lower back and prevents **inactivity** and **stiffness** when you are sitting down.

ROLLING

An action that is performed many times every night when sleeping. Rolling can also be performed as a regular exercise. (See **mobilising exercises**.)

ROTATION

Rotation at any one level of the back is small and the movement should be performed with the whole back acting in synchrony, the **pelvis** and rotation of the **hip** joints playing a large part in helping the back. Rotation is greatest in the **cervical region**, at the pivot joint of the **atlas** and **axis**, allowing the head to turn, with the rotation in the lower **neck** at the bodies and **joints** of the vertebrae C6, C7 and T1. In the **thoracic region**, rotation is limited by the **rib** cage, and it is minimal in the **lumbar region**, because the **facet joints** change direction.

Each small facet joint has to be kept fully mobile, otherwise problems and subsequent damage will occur. You should avoid any forceful **twisting** movements. (See **mobilising exercises**.)

RUGBY

The head-on collisions that occur in rugby, and the **pushing and pulling** that occur in the pack and scrum, are bad for the back unless correct techniques are adopted at an early stage, the **neck** being the most vulnerable area. (See **biomechanics, levers**). **Muscle** and **joint** problems are frequent, often due to tight powerfully bunched muscle tissues which have been specifically built up for power and endurance. (See **exercise, sport**.)

RUNNING

This activity can help increase mobility in the hips, knees and ankles, which will give the back better protection for daily activities. Running on the toes with a springing long stride will minimise the **jarring** on the back. A **rebounding** unit can help the warm up period for running.

Correct footwear should always be worn, and good running **shoes**, with sorbothane cushioning which hold the heel firmly, are essential. The rules and tips for **jogging** also apply for running.

RUPTURED DISC

A herniated or protruding **disc** is often called a ruptured disc.

SACRUM

The broad triangular wedge of bone made up of five fused **vertebrae** situated between the two ilia is called the sacrum. (See **anatomy**.) It lies within the pelvic girdle at the base of the back, and the entire backbone balances on top of it. (See **pelvis**.) It joins the two ilia at the sacroiliac joints. At the tip of the sacrum lies the **coccyx**.

The sacrum is rarely damaged, but the most likely cause would be injury in a car accident.

Sacroiliac joints

The two sacroiliac joints lie on either side of the sacrum, binding it with the two ilia to form the pelvic girdle. They are strong joints, bound back and front by tough **ligaments**, and therefore are relatively difficult to strain compared with the **joints** in the long beanpole back above. It is thought that there is very little movement at these joints; however, movement can occur, especially during **pregnancy**, when hormone activity takes place causing softening and stretching of the ligaments.

Some common causes of sacroiliac injury and strain are:

- A fall on the bottom.
- A **short leg**.
- Pregnancy.
- **Childbirth**.
- Swinging a **golf** club.
- A **twisting** manipulative movement. (See **rotation**.)
- Moving heavy furniture. (See **carrying, lifting**.)
- Digging in the garden. (See **gardening**.)
- Sailing and **windsurfing**.
- A **rugby** scrum injury.

For what to do, see **acute back**, **chronic back**, **corset**, **pelvic tilt**, **posture**.

SAGGING

Don't!

SAUNA

Saunas are popularly associated with Scandinavia, especially Finland. A dry heat is followed by a moist heat, produced by pouring water on heated rocks, and it is this which stimulates the **circulation**. Many people worldwide find relief for minor back problems from taking a sauna. The icy water plunge, which is the third stage of the therapy, is often eliminated, although the contrast can be extremely invigorating for the whole body. Follow the sauna by a **massage** if you can.

SCAR TISSUE

This is the tissue formed in the healing process after inflammatory changes and injury. (See **inflammation**.) It can cause limitation of movement in the back since it does not have the same properties of elasticity as **ligaments** and **muscles**. (See **adhesions, fibrositis**.)

SCHEUERMANN'S DISEASE

This disease is sometimes known as adolescent **kyphosis** or round back, but **osteochondritis** is the medical name now accepted internationally.

Heredity plays a part in its development, but research has not yet established a cause. The condition is fairly common and results in an altered shape to the back, **stiffness** and backache, since the **vertebrae** do not grow symmetrically and become wedge shaped. You should see the **doctor** for **X-rays** and a diagnosis if you suspect this condition is present.

SCHOOLBAGS

Schoolbags and satchels weighed down with heavy books, can cause problems to the growing child, as they are often carried on one shoulder. (See *backache, scoliosis*.) It is therefore important that the weight of books and homework is evenly distributed in a satchel or a rucksack on the back in yoke fashion, across the shoulders like an old-fashioned milkmaid.

You should explain the importance of correct *carrying* and *lifting*, and encourage your child to develop good habits with a good *posture*. Don't allow your child to have a fashionable *bag* unless it can be carried correctly.

SCHOOLCHILDREN

Children sit for many hours a day bent over schoolwork. It is therefore vitally important that parents, teachers and local authorities combine to prevent back problems in the next generation. Children should 'be fit to sit.'

Dr Aage *Mandal* has been a great pioneer in this area. Flat *desk* tops and straight horizontal *chairs* lead to poor sitting postures and incorrect eyesight levels for the blackboard.

Go and look at your child's school – is the furniture good enough for your child's growing back?

SCIATIC NERVE

The sciatic nerve is formed by numerous nerves from the *spinal cord* from the roots of L4, L5, S1 and S2 in the lower back. (See *anatomy, lumbar region, sacrum*.) These nerves combine into one big nerve in the *pelvis*, with branches extending down into the leg.

Sciatica

Sciatica is a common complaint, usually caused by *compression* or a mechanical irritation. It describes the *inflammation* in the sciatic nerve which runs down the back of the leg. The referred *pain*, felt in the buttock, back of the thigh, calf or big toe, is usually due to one of the following causes:

- Sudden stress and *strain* due to falling, *lifting*, pulling or reaching. (See *pushing and pulling*.)
- Pressure of a *disc* which has prolapsed or protruded in the lower back on the sciatic nerve.
- Pinching of the nerve by *osteophytes* which encroach at the facet *joints*. (See *osteoarthritis*.)
- Muscle *spasm* which stretches the nerve sheath and prevents the back from *bending*. (See *scoliosis*.)
- Added strain during *pregnancy*.

If you get sciatica, stop all movements that aggravate the sciatic nerve, such as driving the *car, walking* or *sitting* down. (See *acute back*.)

SCOLIOSIS

Scoliosis is an increased lateral curvature of the back that can cause low back *pain*. There are several causes:

- Severe muscle *spasm* due to carrying school books on one side of the body, carrying heavy *shoulderbags*, too much *shopping* or an overloaded briefcase.
- *Heredity* factors.
- *Congenital* abnormalities.

The lateral curvature in scoliosis results in the *ligaments* becoming overstretched and elongated on one side and shortened and tight on the other side. The *muscles* also become stretched on one side and tight on the other, therefore causing an imbalance. (See *biomechanics*.)

Functional scoliosis

The scoliosis which is ligamentous and has muscular causes is called functional scoliosis.

This is a temporary condition without bony changes in the spine, and the **pelvis** is not level at the anterior superior iliac crests. (See **strain**). It can be corrected by **mobilising exercises, pelvic tilt** exercises, attention to **posture**, and **swimming**.

Structural scoliosis

When the pelvis is level and bony changes in the back are causing a sideways pull, it is known as structural scoliosis. If the causes are due to congenital and bony changes you should see a doctor for **X-rays**, and there should be regular screening tests in the growing child. **Braces** may be necessary to correct the scoliosis. (See **observation**.)

Check your child today.

SEATING

See **chairs, supports**.

SELF HELP

'God helps them that help themselves.'
Benjamin Franklin, 1706–1790

It is YOUR back – YOU are responsible for it. Three out of four people can help themselves get better. (See **acute back**, **chronic back**, **help**, Where to Get Help and Suggested Further Reading.)

SEX

This is often one of the last questions about back problems to be discussed by the medical profession, even though it is sometimes the underlying cause. However, a vigorous sensible sex life can be a great help to a bad back – bedroom Olympics are not a must but, unless you have an extremely painful back or a severe problem, sexual activity is very good for your back.

- Extreme **fatigue** can cause a bad back, so be rested when you have sex, or just refreshingly exhausted.
- Sex will get your blood flowing, increase your oxygen intake and make you feel better. (See **aerobics, circulation**.)
- Sex should be a pleasure, not a painful experience, so if you have a bad back don't try and overcome **pain** by sexual intercourse.
- Find a **position** that suits your back without any discomfort. If in pain, choose whether the top or bottom position is more suitable for your back.
- Let your back problem enhance your sex life rather than limit it. Understand your **anatomy**: don't use it as an excuse for avoiding sex.
- Choose a good **bed**.
- Avoid jerky movements, and try and line up the **pelvis** as you would to achieve good **posture**. (See **jarring, pelvic tilt**.)
- Mobilise and strengthen the lower back muscles. (See **mobilising exercises**.)
- Relax and enjoy it. If you are tense or frightened of a poor performance then don't do it. (See **relaxation, tension**.)

NOTE: Let your partner provide the action if you have a bad back; don't try and prove anything, it won't signal catastrophe. Seek therapy counselling or medical help if you are having problems or if the pain persists for some time. Remember, a little kindness will help, so have lots of tender loving care.

SHIATSU

Shiatsu is a Japanese form of finger **acupressure** that stimulates the reflex points of nerve pathways, rebalancing the body's energy structure and unblocking areas of tension. A shiatsu therapist works on a specific area and its **meridian**, and this can be effective in reducing muscle **tension** and **stress** in the back.

SHOES

Shoes often cause back problems. A shoe should hold the foot well, especially around the heel and over the instep. (See *feet*.) Fashion often dictates the style of shoes, but it will pay dividends if you choose sensible shoes which fit properly; children's growing feet should be measured for shoes every three months:

- High heels can cause tight Achilles tendons, leading to pain in the calves, back and neck.
- Very narrow high heels and shoes with no backs can cause wobbling which causes poor *balance* and excessive muscular activity when *walking* with subsequent backache.
- 'Negative' heeled shoes where the front foot is higher than the heel so the entire shoe slopes backwards from front to rear are also a hazard.
- The shock absorbing qualities of the heels of shoes are important to prevent *jarring* on the back. Crepe rubber soles and heels are best, in fact anything that is bouncy and cushions the spine. Some excellent insoles for shoes are manufactured by *Spenco*.

It is essential that footwear should fit well, with the back of the shoe hugging the heel firmly, otherwise it will ride up and down, you will not be able to walk properly and this will cause further strain on the back.

SHOPPING

Apply the principles of good *lifting* and *carrying* when you are shopping. For example, take care not to bend into the boot of the car when removing shopping from the trolley – use the *pelvic tilt* and the *abdominal muscles* to help you.

Large brown paper sacks, which you carry near your chest, are available at checkout counters and are better for carrying shopping than a variety of carrier *bags* or large heavy boxes which can be unwieldy to lift out of a trolley and which may collapse.

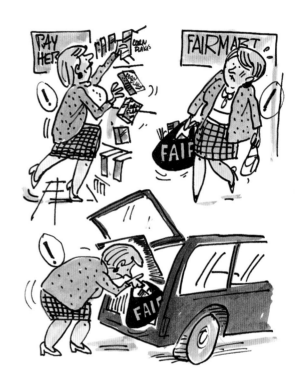

SHORT LEG

Slight variation in leg length is not unusual, and a minimal difference will not cause too many mechanical problems. (See *biomechanics*.) There may be no anatomical difference in the leg length, so it is important to have accurate measurement by a qualified orthopaedic practitioner, as a short leg may only be the result of temporary muscle *spasm* or excessive flexing at the hip joint when walking. (See *orthopaedics*.) An *X-ray* taken in the standing position will establish a short leg.

A shoe raise by a qualified *orthotist* may be necessary and *posture* correction and walking re-education may be necessary from a qualified therapist to balance the *pelvis* and legs.

SHORTWAVE DIATHERMY

This is a form of heat treatment used by physiotherapists to reduce muscle **spasm**. (See **electrotherapy**.)

SHOULDERBAGS

If you must use a shoulderbag, shift the weight from side to side as a heavy bag will cause deviation to one side, **scoliosis** and subsequent back and **neck** ache. Avoid strain wherever possible, and use your strong arm muscles to carry heavy **bags**.

SHOULDERS

The shoulders should be as relaxed as possible for a good **posture**. If there is any tension and you are doing a sedentary job all day and bending forwards, then **mobilising exercises** for the upper shoulders and **neck** will help.

Pain underneath the shoulder blades, called subscapular pain, is a common condition and is usually due entirely to muscle **tension** or referred **pain** from a nerve, radiating from the **thoracic region**. This results in discomfort and pain in the ribs and chest area.

It is important to **warm up** the shoulder girdle as well as the upper back and neck before starting any racquet games such as **badminton**, **tennis** or **squash**.

SHOWERS

If you have an **acute back** it is easier to have a shower than a **bath** – the effect of water jetting on to a painful area of the back will relieve **spasm** and **tension**. Make sure you have a non-slip shower mat.

SITTING

A good sitting **posture** is important at work and during periods of relaxation so you are able to relax and work without pain, stress, strain or fatigue.

Sedentary life = Disuse = Flabby muscles = Backache = Fatigue = Stress.

Tips

- Have a good, properly shaped **chair** for your back.
- The hips and knees should be flexed, with the feet on the floor.
- Accustom your body to moving while sitting. Be dynamic, not static.
- Use **pillows**, and lumbar **supports** in your chair or **car** seat.
- Don't sit with **crossed legs**. A one-sided pull on the spine causes **compression**.
- There must be adequate support of the back so the lumbar **curve** is maintained without muscular effort.

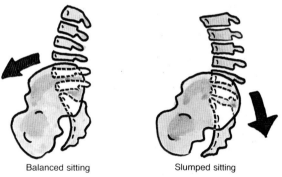

Balanced sitting   Slumped sitting

Sitting at a desk

Have everything – the telephone, paper clips, the stapler – either within easy reach, so you do not have to overstretch, or alternatively put everything at the other side of the room so you have to get up frequently. Use telephone directories if you need an instant footstool.

Sitting in the theatre, cinema and restaurants

Take your lumbar support. Hopefully it will make public places aware that they need better seating!

SIT–UPS

This exercise is very popular with lots of people. It is performed with the legs straight, and the back being raised from a lying position to the sit-up position.

However, sit-ups can be extremely hard on a weak back and should NOT be performed if you have a back problem. Weak **abdominal muscles**, an increased **lordosis** and pain in the hip flexors can be made worse, so until your musculature is really strong, don't do sit-ups.

SKIING

This sport can be hard on the back due to the **twisting, rotation** and turning involved in skiing, and the many falls on the bottom you may have as a beginner. Two or three weeks' training in preparation for skiing can make a big difference to fitness on the slopes. (See **coccydinia sport, warming up**.) The Chartered Society of Physiotherapy will provide an A–Z guide for pre-skiing instruction.

SKIPPING

Skipping, or rope jumping as it is now sometimes called, is a good enjoyable activity – it is simple and will improve your **aerobic** fitness. It will also **tone** the muscles of the arms and legs, but care should be taken not to jar the back by skipping on a hard surface. (See **jarring**.) A rebounder is a suitable piece of apparatus on which to perform skipping exercises. (See **rebounding**.)

SLEEPING

Are you getting enough sleep, or are you tired, with a sagging slouched back?

What to do

- Buy a good **bed**.
- Have enough **pillows** for good support.
- Keep warm in bed.
- Vary your **position**, and don't sleep on your stomach if you have a bad back unless you have a pillow under the hips to avoid over-**extension**.
- If you sleep on your back, put a pillow under your knees.
- If you sleep on your side, bend at the hips and knees and use pillows where necessary.
- Don't lie still for too long; roll over and turn whenever possible.
- Don't leap out of bed when the alarm goes. Set it five minutes before you need to get up and stretch gently in bed first.
- Ankle rotation exercises first thing in the morning and last thing at night will maintain **circulation** and may prevent cramps.

Sleep any way that is comfortable.

SLINGS

Back pain is one of the common factors which affects anyone who has to lift or handle a patient. The MeDesign handling sling, which was conceived and designed by Dr Duncan Troup, is a simple and widely used aid to reduce the load on the back when **lifting** a heavy patient. The sling works by making the arms effectively longer. You do not have to bend so far forward to reach under the patient. (See **bending**.) The back is thus kept more upright and, by avoiding **twisting**,

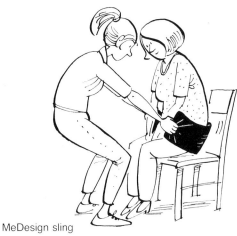

MeDesign sling

there is maximum mechanical advantage to help you in the lift. (See **biomechanics**.) Slings can also be useful when lifting a person up onto the bed or during transfer from the bed to a chair or when standing.

SLIPPED DISC

This term is incorrect. The **disc** does not slip, it protrudes or bulges. (See **disc**.)

SMILE

Smile! It's good for you.

SMOKING

Smoking is bad for your general health and therefore bad for your back.

SNEEZING

When your back and body are suddenly thrown forwards as you sneeze, it jerks the back and causes pain. A **facet joint** may then become locked or jammed. (See **jamming, locking**.) Therefore, it you feel you are going to sneeze:

- Tighten your **abdominal muscles** as you are thrown forwards, to prevent flying backwards suddenly.
- Bend your **knees** slightly.
- Relax slowly and control your **breathing** to prevent further sneezing. (See **relaxation**.)

SOFAS

Avoid soft saggy sofas and stretching forward to reach low coffee tables. Sit on the floor instead. (See **chairs, furniture**.)

SOMMELIER

The **pillow** from Sommelier incorporates the principle of the oriental neck roll used extensively in the Far East. It is made of three sections; a middle section and two symmetrical sides. The two slightly higher and firmer sides support the head and neck while lying on either side of the body, while the middle section is lower and designed to accommodate the head and neck while lying on the back.

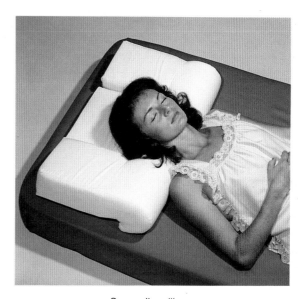

Sommelier pillow

SPASM

When **muscles** lose the ability to relax, and stay in a sustained contraction as a continued involuntary action, it is called muscle spasm. Spasm will lead to tenderness and eventually wasting if it is allowed to continue and muscles will be painful under pressure. (See **acute back** for what to do.)

Causes of muscle spasm

- Weak muscles.
- Cold **draughts**. (See **air conditioning**.)
- Emotional **tension**. (See **emotions**.)
- **Disc** prolapse.
- An injury.

SPENCER

See **Flexfit**.

SPENCO

Spenco Medical was established by Dr W. Spence during the late 1960s. A specialist in physical medicine and rehabilitation, Dr Spence set about developing an elastomer that could be used to recreate the properties of the fatty layers of the skin and absorb shock and vibration. Today Spenco supplies neoprene supports and insoles for the feet and **hot wraps** and **cold wraps** for use in the treatment of the back. (See **cold therapy, heat therapy, shoes**.)

SPINAL CORD

The spinal cord – a thick bundle of nerves – is connected to the **brain** at the top, and travels from the head, like a telephone cable, to the second lumbar **vertebrae**, where it divides to supply the lower limbs through the vertebral foramina in the **lumbar region** and sacrum. (See **anatomy, nervous system**.)

It is protected inside the spinal canal by six layers:

- The back **muscles**.
- The **ligaments** which keep the vertebrae in place.
- A layer of **fat**.
- The dural membrane, which is the outer membrane enveloping the brain and spinal cord. (See **dura**.)
- A fluid called cerebrospinal fluid.
- Two thin sheaths around the cord itself.

Thirty-one pairs of nerves responsible for muscular control extend from the spinal cord.

SPINE

The spine is the backbone of the body. (See **anatomy**.)

SPINESEAT

See **chairs**.

SPINOUS PROCESS

At the rear of a **vertebra** is a spinous process. These bony outgrowths can be felt when you run your fingers down the centre of the back. (See **transverse processes**.)

SPONDYLOLISTHESIS

This is a difficult word to spell and say! It is the forward displacement of one vertebra on another, and usually occurs at the two lower lumbar **vertebrae**. (See **lumbar region**.) The displacement is an inherent weakness in the back, which occurs gradually during development; once you are fully grown it stops. It can be so slight you may never know you have it, and it will only show up on an **X-ray**. A violent injury or strain during excessive activity will then loosen the already weakened tissues, such as in a **bowler's back**.

If you have spondylolisthesis, back pain is worse when you stand, as in standing it will be aggravated by the lumbar **lordosis**.
NOTE AND WARNING: People with this condition are extremely flexible, but if they intend taking up **ballet** or gymnastics it is as well to spot it in early life. **Pregnant** women are also monitored for this condition.

SPONDYLOSIS

Spondylosis is degeneration of the intervertebral **discs** which also affects the bodies of the **vertebrae**. It is most common in the lower **neck**, mid-**thoracic region** and the lower **lumbar region**, and it causes intermittent pain and restriction of movement. On **X-ray** there is a narrowing of the disc spaces and there are often **osteophytes** present.

There is often confusion between spondylosis and **osteoarthrosis**. Spondylosis affects the vertebral bodies and discs, whereas **osteoarthrosis** affects the **facet joints**. There is **inflammation** in both conditions, but spondylosis tends to occur in the 35–50 age group whereas osteoarthrosis occurs more in the elderly.

What to do

- Rest. (See **acute back**, **positions**.)
- Wear a neck **collar** to support the head. (See **cervical spondylosis**.)
- A **corset** will help support the lumbar region.
- Seek professional medical advice about treatment.

SPORT

Sport is good for heart and lung function and a great way to release emotional tension, compete and have fun. However, many sports are a hazard for the back.

You need to be agile, balanced and mobile for sport. Choose your sport carefully and if you have a bad back think twice before you play **squash**, **tennis**, **rugby**, go **windsurfing** or **parachuting**. (See **agility**, **balance**, **mobilising exercises**.)

Some causes of back pain from sport:

- Lack of warm-ups. (See **warming up**.)
- No **training** schedule.
- Poor **muscle tone**.
- Sloppy technique.
- Starting again too quickly after an injury.
- Trying to keep up competitively.

Simple rules to help your back

- Be fit for your individual sport.
- Warm up and cool down thoroughly.
- Use the right equipment for you, and the right technique.
- Don't overtrain. It is quality rather than quantity that is needed for sport.
- If you have influenza or any other viral infection, don't train.
- See your teacher, a professional expert or watch yourself on a video if you are having trouble with technique – for example a **golf** swing, or a **tennis** backhand.

SPRAIN

The soft tissues such as **ligaments, tendons** or **muscles** are torn when you sprain the back. (See **tear**.) The capsule of a **facet joint** can also be damaged. Acute **inflammation** occurs and the back can be extremely painful. This may result in:

- **Scoliosis** as a result of over-contraction of the muscles which are protecting the affected area.
- **Disc** rupture.
- The collection of fluid in the tissues as a result of the injury, which can lead to the formation of **scar tissue**.
- Muscular **spasm**, which can cause joint imbalance.

What to do

See **acute back**. Be patient; sprains can take a long time to heal. However, see the doctor if the pain has not begun to subside after 48 hours.

SQUASH

This **sport** involves a lot of rapid, unpredictable and contorted movements, so it is not ideal for the back, especially if you are tall. Remember it is extremely competitive, so find a partner at your own level, and do regular **knee** exercises and **squatting** movements whilst **warming up**.

SQUATTING

Stand with your feet shoulder-width apart and tilt

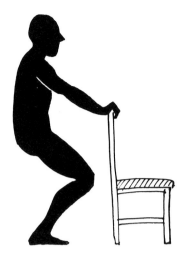

This movement puts very little stress on the back as most of the body weight is taken by the thighs, legs and pelvis. It is a useful position for a lot of activities especially:

- **Lifting**.
- Sitting on the **toilet**.
- As a delivery position for **childbirth**.

STANDING

Standing can cause backache especially if:

- You have to stand for prolonged periods.
- You have poor **posture**.
- Your **pelvic tilt** is incorrect.
- The lower back has an excessive **lordosis**.
- You continually stand on one leg like a stork or a ballet dancer.
- You wear high heels all the time. (See **shoes**.)
- Your **balance** is poor.
- You are tired from lack of **rest** and **sleep**.
- You have a military stance. (See **posture**.)
- You have a **chronic backache**.

your **pelvis** into the correct position. (See **pelvic tilt**.) Use the back of a chair to hold on to for this exercise if your balance is poor. Have your feet in line with the hips so there is a stable base. The knees should be in line with the feet and the hips and knees should be flexible.

Slowly bend at the knees, keeping the back straight until you are squatting. If you have stiff joints, just go as far as your knees will allow without causing any pain. Stand up slowly, pushing with your thigh muscles until you are standing erect. Repeat five times.

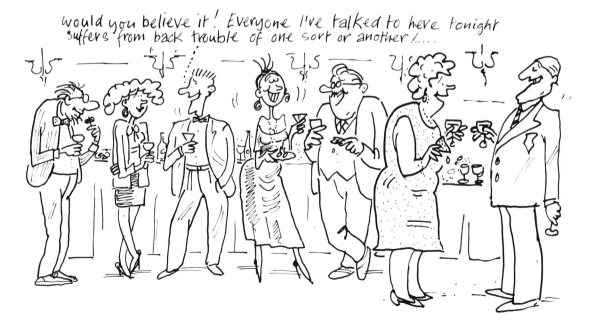

would you believe it! Everyone I've talked to here tonight suffers from back trouble of one sort or another!....

What to do

- Don't stand when you can walk. Standing still for prolonged periods causes the muscles to tire and then you start to slouch. (See *walking*.)
- Check your posture and pelvic tilt continually, using a mirror. Your weight should be evenly distributed on both the feet and hips, in a line just in front of the ankle joint.
- The *feet* should be slightly apart for a stable base, and the body and back relaxed.
- The *knees* should be straight, but not locked.
- Relax the *shoulders*.
- Avoid standing in a bent or stooped position.
- Use a foot stool for one foot if you have to stand for long periods such as *ironing* or in the *pub*. (See *housework*.)

'Stand tall, walk tall.'

STENOSIS

When there is an abnormal constriction or narrowing of the spinal canal it is known as spinal stenosis.

STIFFNESS

Stiffness causes *backache*, and extreme stiffness is very painful. It is caused by fluid collecting in the tissues, resulting in a loss of movement, so it is important to move the back whenever possible, slowly and gently at first, until you can progress to further mobility. (See *extension*, *flexion*, *mobilising exercises*.)

'Keep active, keep moving.'

Morning stiffness

This occurs as a result of:

- A saggy *bed*, a mattress being too soft or poor *pillow positions*.

- An excessive intake of fluid the night before.
- Sleeping pills, which prevent movement during sleep.
- Suddenly taking up a new activity for which the *muscles* do not have enough preparation. (See *tone, warming up*.)
- Overuse of the back the day before.

What to do

Stiffness can be extremely painful, so *exercises* and stretching, especially on waking, are essential to alleviate the stagnation of *circulation* that has occurred during a night's sleep. Ankle rotation exercises and performing the *pelvic tilt* before you get out of bed will help, followed by mobilising exercises.

STRAIN

Muscle and *ligament* strains are very common and are a nuisance since they cause backache. They occur when excessive repetitive *tension* and *stress* are experienced by the back. (See *biomechanics*.)

Since there is a limit to what the back can do, it is found that occupational hazards which involve incorrect *bending* and *lifting* techniques are the usual cause of back strain. A strain begins with an immediate sharp pain which gradually becomes a dull ache, with local tenderness persisting like toothache. The *inflammation* is much milder than with a *sprain* and movements do not become very limited, so you tend to continue with what you are doing.

STOP immediately, and the strain will resolve itself fairly quickly. Otherwise the acute strain will become a *chronic back* problem and might even lead to a sprain.

(See *acute back*, *chronic back* for 'What to do'.)

STRENGTHENING

When your back is free from pain and fully mobile, go to a recognised gym or see a qualified exercise therapist for strengthening **exercises** which are tailored to your requirements. (See **gym**, **Norsk Sequence Training Machines**, **Tunturi** and Where to Get Help.)

STRESS

Stress should be avoided as it can be a hazard for the back.

Mechanical stress

This occurs when there is a breakdown in the functional activity of a **disc**, usually due to overloading and **repetitive movements** which lead to a prolapsed disc. This will affect all the surrounding structures of the back and the stress will show as muscle **spasm** and **pain**.

Psychological stress

Anxiety, tiredness, worry and **fatigue** can all bring about stress. Emotional tension and headaches occur, and the autonomic **nervous system** comes into play, resulting in muscle spasm, a reaction in the internal organs and agony in the back.

What to do

- Be positive about your physical and mental health.
- Keep calm and learn **breathing**, **relaxation** and **yoga** techniques.
- Build up your endurance, but try not to overwork, get tired or become too competitive. (See **aerobics**, **exercise**, **posture**, **sport**.)
- Make your **work** more efficient. (See **ergonomics**, **housework**, **office**.)
- Delays or obstacles beyond your control should encourage you to think about your lifestyle and set achievable goals.
- Have a **rest** or a **holiday**.
- Learn to say no without feeling guilty.
- Make time to see family and friends.
- Smile and laugh.
- If you need help, seek it.

These factors will all help remove stress. However, a certain degree of stress is necessary to stimulate you, and you may even thrive on it. Learn to distinguish between stress and distress.

STRETCHING

Stretching is part of the natural daily routine. Like all animals, stretching and relaxing are essential if you have been in one position for too long, but take care not to overstretch. Stretching will help maintain the **elasticity** of the back, but control your stretches out of any kinked position and do plenty of gentle stretches in a warm-up routine before **gardening**, playing **sport** or **dancing**. (See **warming up**.)

SUITCASES

Always carry two smaller suitcases rather than one large heavy one. (See **carrying, lifting**.) Use a **trolley** or get a porter to help you whenever possible, especially if you have a weak back.

SUPPORTS

Corsets, **collars**, **girdles**, **braces**, lumbar back rests are all supports that are sometimes necessary to help a bad back. But corsets and collars, for example, need to be fitted by a qualified practitioner. You should be taught how to put them on and when to wear them, as **muscles** will become wasted if you rely on them too much. Do not be afraid to ask for simple directions.

There are supports which have been specifically designed for the back.

MCKENZIE ROLLS

Cervical and Lumbar Rolls have been designed by Robin **McKenzie** to support the neck and low back region. They are made of foam and are not more than 3½ to 5 inches (9 – 12½ cm) in diameter before being compressed. They can be placed horizontally to give extra support to the **neck** whilst sleeping and to produce the correct lumbar **curve** when reading, watching television or driving a car. (See **lumbar region**.) A Night Roll is also available which offers support around the waist when you are in a sleeping **position**.

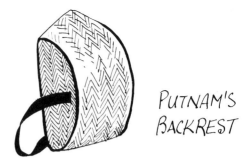

PUTNAM'S BACKREST

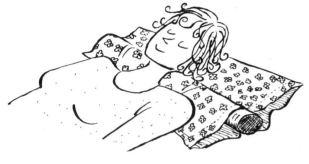

McKenzie Cervical Roll

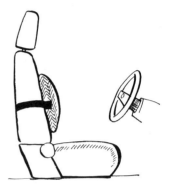

Putnam's backrest used in a car

PUTNAM'S BACKREST

This well-researched and tested support, designed by James **Putnam**, is made of a flame retardant contoured foam on a solid base, covered in a washable material. It is placed in the hollow of the lower back and can be adjusted up or down for maximum comfort and support and then fixed by a strap.

It comes in two sizes. The large model is ideal for the **car**, the home and **office** seating. (See **chairs, workplace**.) The compact model is useful if space is restricted when travelling by coach, train or plane. An inflatable compact travel pillow is also available for supporting the **neck**. (See **air travel**.)

NOTE: Whenever possible, make sure the lumbar support is placed in the area of the back which is correct for your individual problem. See also MeDesign Backfriend in **chairs**.

SURGEONS

Surgeons are the experts who will operate on the back, for example if a **laminectomy**, a **fusion** of the spine, a repair, or the removal of a tumour is necessary. Seventy per cent of back pain sufferers are referred on to a surgeon by their family doctor, but it is seldom necessary to have an operation.

SWAY BACK

See **lordodis**.

SWELLING

See **inflammation**.

SWIMMING

When swimming, the effect of *gravity* on the back is eliminated so there is less *compression* on the *discs* and it is easier to mobilise the back. If your back muscles are weak, swimming is an excellent activity.

It is a good idea to start slowly by floating on the back and trying gentle arm and leg paddling movements. Make sure the water is warm enough, otherwise muscle *spasm* can occur; for example lying on an airbed in the cold sea after sunbathing is a hazard.

Swimming on your front should be discouraged if arching backwards, as in the breaststroke, increases back pain due to the effort of holding the *neck* and head out of the water. Gentle rhythmical strokes, as performed for *hydrotherapy* are the answer. (See Suggested Further Reading and Health Hydros in the Where to Get Help section.)

SYMPATHETIC NERVOUS SYSTEM

This is another name for the autonomic *nervous system*.

SYNOVIAL FLUID

This light slippery fluid lubricates the *joint* surfaces and is found in the *facet joint* spaces of the back.

TABLES

It is important to have a table at the correct height for the **chair** on which you are going to sit, for all activities. (See **ergonomics**.) It is especially important during schooldays when the back is growing – an old-fashioned school **desk** with a sloping top is preferable to a flat-top table. Tilting tables or **writing slopes**, which can accommodate any angle for working, are useful as the sloping surface will reduce the distance between your **eyes** and your work and prevent **bending** and poor **posture**.

TAIL BONE

See **coccyx**.

TEAR

Tearing a **disc, muscle** or **ligament** happens when the fibres or soft tissues are stretched beyond their normal range by force. The back is caught unawares by the sudden movement and, before the muscles can prevent it, a painful tear results with subsequent **inflammation** and muscle **spasm**. (See **acute back** for 'What to do'.)

TEETH

Brushing your teeth is an essential daily task, but can be a hazard for the back. Use an electric toothbrush to shorten the time needed for brushing the teeth, and bend your **knees** or squat if you have to do it over a basin. (See **squatting**.)

TEETH GRINDING

Teeth grinding usually occurs quite subconsciously, but both this and clenching the teeth can cause joint problems in the **neck**, and sometimes **migraine**. See your dentist and the doctor for help.

TELEPHONE

Holding a telephone tightly can lead to **neck** ache and back problems. It will cause **shoulder** and neck **pain** if it is cradled between the neck and the shoulder, and holding two telephones is worse! (See **posture, tension**.) If you find yourself in this position, stop immediately if you want to avoid back problems.

TELEVISION

Sitting watching the television is a hazard. Keep moving at regular intervals, and make sure you have good back **support**. (See **chairs**.)

TEMPERATURE

It is important for the back to be in a constant temperature, otherwise muscle **spasm** will result. (See **air conditioning, draughts**.) Warm clothes will keep the back warm and protect it from the cold. During sleep, the body temperature drops so make sure that the blankets or duvet cover the neck and shoulders and the lower back is not exposed. (See **bedding**.) Lying on an airbed in a cool sea after sunbathing can cause severe muscle spasm.

TENDON

A tendon is a very tough fibrous band which joins one end of a **muscle** to a **bone**. Tendons have their own blood and nerve supply, so are able to repair themselves and also to distinguish **pain**.

TENNIS

Tennis is a repetitive game, using the same muscles for the same movements, such as serving and hard volley smashes. (See *repetitive movements*.) The long leverage of the racquet when you go to stretch for a ball can easily wrench the back. (See *levers*.) Also, the continual jumping about on hard courts to spring for a ball can cause unnecessary *jarring* of the back.

If you have a bad back:

- Try table tennis instead.
- *Exercise* the *muscles* on the other side of the body.
- Wear a lumbar *support*.
- If you must play, do it gently on a grass court.

TENSION

Back *pain* can be induced by both mental and physical tension, so it is important to ask yourself whether you had tension before the back trouble, or vice versa.

Causes of tension

- Poor *posture* as as result of a recent injury, *muscle spasm* or *stiffness*.
- Hard work without any *holiday*, *rest* or *relaxation* leading to *stress*.
- Extreme *fatigue* and lack of sleep.
- *Anger*, *anxiety* and worry.
- An unsatisfying *sex* life.

What to do

- Learn to understand your *emotions*.
- Identify *anger* and *anxiety*.
- Programme your work routine so subconsciously you don't become aggravated or tired.
- Use *ergonomics* to design your *workplace*.

- Have frequent *massage* sessions.
- Learn *breathing* exercises.
- Go to *relaxation* classes.
- See a psychologist for help if you really need it.
- Talk to the family and friends – 'a trouble shared is a trouble halved.'

THALASSO THERAPY

Taking the waters has been popular for thousands of years, with the Romans, the French, the Germans and the Swiss. Thalasso therapy, which is derived from the Greek *thalassa*, meaning sea, is based on the concept that elements such as iodine, magnesium, calcium and sulphur are lacking in people who are run down, and can be absorbed by the body through the skin.

Seawater contains these and other essential substances. It is hosed at the body, envigorating the *circulation*, revitalising the tissues and stimulating the *nervous system.*

THERAPY

The effectiveness of any therapy depends on a good match between both the client and the type of therapy which is being used, and the client and the therapist. A therapist cannot help a client who feels ill at ease because of a mismatch in personalities or therapy techniques. There are several ways to find a therapist (see Where To Get Help section at the end of the book.) Ask about qualifications, registration, techniques and, of course, fees.

'If it's physical, it's therapy.'

THERMAL

Thermal clothing is a great help in keeping the back warm in cold weather, especially for elderly people. (See *temperature*.)

THIGHS

The thighs or upper part of the legs are especially important for **lifting**. The **muscles** that form the thigh help all back movements and they should be especially strong to lift the body weight and to avoid injury. (See **hamstrings, knees, quadriceps**.)
NOTE: **Walking** is excellent for these muscles.

THORACIC REGION

This is the chest or trunk region of the back. It is the longest section consisting of 12 **vertebrae**, numbered T1 to T12. (See **anatomy**.) Each vertebrae forms a special **joint** as it articulates with two **ribs**; the ribs come off each side and encircle the chest, forming the ribcage and joining up with the breastbone, the sternum, in the front. The ribcage protects the heart and lungs.
   The thoracic region is relatively immobile. It is involved in the movements of the ribcage concerned with **breathing**.

TIGHTNESS

A common cause of pain in the back is a pull on tight structures. Tight back **muscles** and **hamstrings**, which run along the back of the **thighs** to just below the **knee**, will make **bending** forwards difficult and painful.

TIME

'Time is the physician.'
Benjamin Disraeli, 1804–1881

TINGLING

A tingling sensation is felt when there is pressure on a nerve; if it is allowed to continue, the area will become painful. If numbness then follows, the nerve has been completely cut off, so it is important to release the pressure as soon as you feel any tingling. (See **compression**.)

TIREDNESS

If you feel worn out and generally very tired, it can cause backache. Slow down and get plenty of **rest** and **sleep**.

TODDLER

See **babies** and **children**.

TOILETS

When sitting on the toilet, it is important to:

- Sit upright, resting the feet on a low footstool. This helps to bring the knees slightly higher than the hips and avoids hurting the back.
- Try not to bend forwards, with your tummy muscles sagging loosely in front. (See **abdominal muscles**.)
- Learn how to **squat**.
- Avoid constipation, since any increase in pressure within the abdomen during bowel movement will cause nerve irritation and **tension**.
- Have a high lavatory seat.

The address of the Disabled Living Foundation is in the Where To Get Help section; they will be able to advise where to get equipment.

TOMOGRAPHY

See **CAT scan**.

TONE

Tone describes the feeling of a contraction in a **muscle**. The greater the tone, the less the muscle is able to extend. Muscle tone is important in holding the bones in the correct relative positions to provide good **posture** and **balance**.

TORTICOLLIS

See *whiplash*.

TOUCH

All manual therapists use touch – one of the oldest healing arts. Not only can it be physically relaxing, but touch with the fingers can tell the therapist about the state of the back and its tissues, sensitive spots and the presence of *tension*. Learn to touch, and have regular *massage* to ease tight structures and tired muscles.

TRACTION

Traction can be a great relief for a painful back, especially where *disc* symptoms are present. It pulls the joints of the back apart to release pressure.

- Hang from a door or bar and allow the weight of the legs to exert a traction force on the back. Relax all the muscles of the back and legs and allow the dead weight to pull the *vertebrae* apart. The hands gripping the top of the door will tire quite quickly, but it is a method you can do at home. (See *hanging*.)

- Traction can be given in bed or on an electrically operated table under supervision in *hospital* or by a registered qualified practitioner in a treatment room. A *corset* is applied around the *pelvis* and another band around the trunk. A system of pulleys and weights provide the traction, and it may be sustained, intermittent or rhythmic, according to the back symptoms.

- For cervical or *neck* traction only, a halter is applied to the head and neck with cords and a spreader. Such traction can be given manually or mechanically, while seated or lying down, and it is thought to be safer than *manipulation*, providing it is applied correctly.

- Traction can be given manually using the body weight of the patient and the pull and body weight of the medical practitioner.

- A piece of apparatus called the *Trapeze* can also be used at home, but with initial advice from a medical practitioner.

- Another form of traction which can be used at home is *inversion* therapy.

NOTE: Traction should never be given without an *X-ray* first, to confirm the *diagnosis*.

TRAINING

If you intend to undergo some rigorous activity or *sport* it is important to train properly, to avoid *strains* and *sprains* of the back. A good exercise training programme should be planned so that you are fit for your event, match, or game. Competitive sport such as *tennis*, *rugby*, *golf* or *squash* can produce back pain so plenty of warm ups and a regular training programme are important to keep you fit and supple. (See *warming up*.) It is best to train with an instructor who specialises in the sport, or write to the particular sports association for a programme of exercises.

TRANQUILLISERS

These may be prescribed for back pain as they have some muscle relaxant properties and can help emotional *tension* in an acute episode. (See *drugs*.)

TRANSCUTANEOUS NERVE STIMULATION

Transcutaneous electrical nerve stimulation (TENS) is given by the application of an electrical current from a 9-volt battery through tiny electrodes attached to the skin. The current travels via a nerve root to the central **nervous system**, relieving the pain production in that nerve. The electrical current stimulates the release of **endorphins**.

TENS is applied at one of the following:

- **Trigger points** in the painful region.
- **Acupuncture** points.
- The route of the nerve in the painful area.

The treatment will take 15–20 minutes. You can even use TENS at home; it is quite safe, unless you have a pacemaker or are pregnant, but you should learn how to use it from a qualified medical practitioner, and check on the contraindications before you have this treatment.

TRANSVERSE PROCESSES

From the bony arch round the spinal canal, the transverse processes protrude at the sides of the vertebral bodies. (See **spinal cord**, **vertebra**.)

TRAPEZE

This piece of apparatus is a portable traction unit, designed and developed by a Dutch physiotherapist, Kees Bruin. It is based on the **flexion** technique, that is full 90-degree flexion of the knees and hips. The unit is compact and simple to operate, making it suitable for home use. The traction is manually self operated, has few moving components and no electric hazards. The product has the advantage of being easily

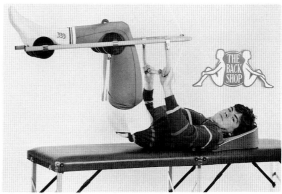
The Trapeze

activated, thus quickly relieving pain, providing an ideal relaxed position and restoring confidence. (See **traction**.)

TRAVEL

Tips for travelling

- Place one or two small **pillows**, a **McKenzie** lumbar roll or use a **Putnam's** Backrest or a MeDesign Backfriend in the lumbar curve of the back when travelling by road, rail or air. (See **cars**, **chairs**, **supports**.)
- If you are short and your feet do not touch the ground, put a piece of small luggage or a book under your feet. (See **sitting**.)
- In a **car**, stop every half hour for a walk if you have backache; in an aeroplane or on a train, walk up and down the aisle. Tall long-legged people should ask for seats where they can stretch their legs, near an emergency exit or on an aisle seat. (See **air travel**, **walking**.)
- Rest your hands and arms on a **pillow** placed on your lap to help **neck** and **shoulder** problems.
- If you have had a back condition, remember to take a **collar** and a **corset** in your suitcase in case you may need them. Wear a corset or a collar to avoid excessive **jarring** from braking or a poor landing if you have to travel with an **acute back** or **chronic back** problem.
- Spread the weight of any luggage you may

have to carry and use a **trolley** or a **suitcase** on wheels where possible.

- If you have a bad back and arrive **jet lagged** at your destination, have a hot **bath** and go to bed.
- If your back is in acute **pain**, do NOT travel.

TREATMENT

See the Where To Get Help section at the end of the book for where to get treatment for the back from professional organisations and other sources.

TRIGGER POINTS

Trigger points are small painful tender areas which you can feel with your fingertips. These **nodules** of **inflammation** can literally trigger off **pain** and muscle **spasm**. Spasm may be present around a trigger point or it may arise as a result of pressing a trigger point. (See **acupuncture, fibrositis, transcutaneous nerve stimulation**.)

TROLLEYS

Trolleys are extremely helpful for **carrying shopping**, dustbins, luggage and **lifting** other heavy objects, but make sure the load is transferred correctly from a trolley to the place of destination.

TUBERCULOSIS

This disease can occur in the spine, although preventative measures mean it is now a very rare condition.

TUMOUR

Any growth or tissue enlargement in the back which causes pain will have to be investigated and perhaps removed by **surgery**.

TUNTURI

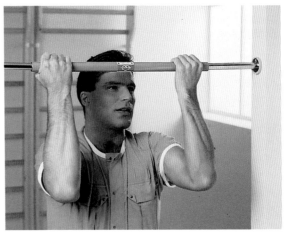

Tunturi exercise bar

TUNTURI

Tunturi of Finland are one of the most experienced manufacturers of **gym** equipment in the world; through years of research, development and design, as well as collaboration with doctors and research workers, they have developed a range of products supported by high technology and extensive testing. Smooth, safe exercise for the whole family is the philosophy behind Tunturi exercise and fitness equipment.

These factors make the Tunturi exercise cycles and rowers excellent for home or professional gyms, and their exercise bar will assist strengthening exercises for the back. (See gym equipment in Where to Get Help at the back of the book for details of distributors.)

TWISTING

Fierce twisting movements – for example, disco dancing and the violent **rotation** movements that are sometimes in fashion for dancing – can lead to **disc** and **joint** problems. However, gentle twisting movements will improve mobility, relaxing and stretching the lower back and pelvic region. (See **mobilising exercises**.)

UGLY

'Though ugliness be the opposite of beauty
It is not the opposite to proportion and fitness'
Edmund Burke, 1729–1797

ULTRASONOGRAPHY

Diagnostic **ultrasound** is used in some medical centres to measure the diameter of the spinal canal by timing the echo produced by an ultrasonic beam. It is not painful – in fact it uses the same principle as an ultrasound scan during pregnancy. (See **spinal cord**.)

ULTRASOUND

An **electrotherapy** treatment which helps in the alleviation of back pain, especially in the acute phase. The high-frequency sound waves vibrate deep in the tissues, agitate the cells and, by increasing the **circulation**, produce heat. The head of the machine is moved constantly to prevent damage to the tissues. It should always be applied by a qualified registered practitioner. (See **physiotherapy**.)

USEFUL PRODUCTS

There are many useful products which can help in the prevention of back problems and provide support when it is necessary:

- Backfriend (see **chairs**).
- Balans Pendulum (see **chairs**).
- Balans Tripos (see **chairs**).
- Bay Jacobsen Mattress Topper (see **beds**).
- **Bed** boards.
- Cold Wrap (see **cold therapy**).
- **Copyholder**.
- Credo **chair**.
- Ergoform **chair**.
- **Flexfit** support.
- Hot Wrap (see **hot therapy**).
- Labomatic working **chair**.
- McKenzie Cervical, Lumbar and Night Rolls (see **McKenzie, supports**).
- 'Mind Your Back' video.
- **Norsk sequence training equipment**.
- Partners **beds**.
- **Pro-Pil-o** pillows.
- **Putnam's** Backrest (see **supports**).
- **Slings**.
- **Sommelier**.
- Spine Seat **chairs**.
- **Trapeze**.
- **Tunturi**.
- **Waterbeds**.
- Wedge (see **Putnam**).
- Woolrest Sleeper (see **beds**).
- **Writing slope**.

UTERUS

A large retroverted uterus, or womb, may cause back **pain** or a dull ache. When the uterus is retroverted, the top part, instead of tilting towards the abdomen, tips the other way. The strain of this tilt may cause pain, and as a result it may be necessary to remove the uterus by a hysterectomy. (See **gynaecology**.)

VARICOSE VEINS

When selecting a **chair**, it is important to choose one that does not aggravate the veins in the legs. Crossing the legs, which always seems to occur when seated on a bad chair, is terrible for the alignment of the back and even worse for the veins. (See **circulation**, **crossed legs**.)

VERTEBRAE

The backbone is composed of 24 individual vertebrae stacked on top of one another, with **discs** in between, and nine fused vertebrae. (See **anatomy**.) Each vertebra can move a little in relation to the ones above and below, making the back a flexible column.

Vertebrae are strong resilient bones which are made to last a lifetime. A typical vertebra has a body, a neural arch and seven processes or projections. The front of each vertebra is solid **bone**, the body of the vertebra. To the sides and rear of each vertebra are a number of bony projections, called the spinous and **transverse processes**. These support the **muscles** which, with the vertebrae, allow for flexibility and movement of the back. Other processes act as hinges in the form of **joints** which interlock the vertebral column. Behind the bodies of each vertebra the bone forms an arch, a central canal, that runs in tube-like fashion down the entire length of the back, from the head to the tail, forming a protective channel. It contains the nerves of the **spinal cord** and is known as the spinal canal.

VIBRATION

Truck and tractor driving, powerboat racing and the vibration in some low-slung racing-type cars can cause back pain. The juddering effect on the spine, with continual vibration over a period of time, abuses the *discs* and *joints*. (See **jarring**.)

VIBRATORY THERAPY

There are several products on the market offering **massage** and **pain** relief by vibratory motorised pads. In order to aid **circulation** and provide a minor improvement of muscle *tone*, they should operate at more than 50 cycles per second for 15–20 minutes at any one time. Care should be taken not to buy an expensive piece of gadgetry which has not passed the recognised equipment standards, so it is wise to consult a medical practitioner for advice before investing in a machine that offers vibration but which may do your back more harm than good. (See **electrotherapy**.)

VIDEO CASSETTES

There are many excellent video presentations which give you information about the back. They are a constant reminder of how to prevent back problems, how to lift correctly, how to get in and out of bed, how to get in and out of a chair, and give advice on exercises and posture. (See **useful products** and Where to Get Help.)

VIGOUR

The activity and strength of your mind and body are essential if you are to preserve an energetic lifestyle. But don't be over vigorous when you are recovering from an illness, as it may cause back problems. Regular **exercise** in moderation improves vigour.

VIOLENT MOVEMENT

The back does not like violent movement. (See **jarring, vibration**.)

VISUAL DISPLAY UNIT (VDU)

After the conventional desk, with typewriter, telephone, notes and books, the VDU is perhaps the most common piece of equipment found in industry or any *office* today. However, working at a VDU can strain the *eyes*, the *nervous system* and alter the *posture* of the back.

There are several controversial views about what to do, which type of chair is most suitable and whether the keyboard should be at elbow level or not. The best advice is to do what is most comfortable and suitable for your back, as no two individuals have the same requirements. If necessary get specialist advice.

Suggestions

- Have a *chair* with easy-to-touch controls for the back support.
- The seat should tilt forwards. (See *Balans*.)
- Have a movable back support which is *ergonomically* designed to follow your movements from the upright position to the forward tilting positions.
- Make sure that the height adjustment of the chair fits you and the *desk* on which the VDU is placed, and that there is full mobility at all angles.
- A waterfall seat will prevent pressure on the thighs, which will help the *circulation*.
- Have adjustable arm supports to prevent *neck* and *shoulder* strain.
- Look slightly down at the VDU screen. If the head is tipped up it will cause *tension* in the head, neck and shoulders.
- Do not tip the head down too much, as this will also cause *strain* in the back.
- Avoid *sitting* too long at the VDU. Get up and walk around.
- If you find you are having muscle *strain*, the unit may be too close or too far away.
- Have your *eyes* tested regularly if you use a VDU every day.

- It is important to have no direct source of lighting, especially one that may reflect on the screen.
- Use a *copyholder* with an adjustable height so that you can position the paper at the right height and angle.

VITALITY

'If a body has vitality enough to be alive under the wrong conditions, it has vitality enough to get well under right conditions, in the absence of serious organic breakdown.'

W.D. Hay, MD

VITAMINS

Vitamins and minerals keep the body efficient and help avoid weakness by playing a major role in building and replacing worn out cells in the *bones* and tissues. For example, calcium is essential for the upkeep of bones, since the mineral is one of the chief constituents of bone; muscle *tone* too partly depends on an adequate supply of calcium in the bloodstream and soft tissue fluids. Calcium tablets can be used to augment our intake from food sources, but make sure that you take a preparation that is easily absorbed.

However, of equal importance in this respect is vitamin D, produced by the action of sunlight on the skin and found in dairy products, eggs and especially fish oils. Vitamin D is thought to increase the absorption of *calcium* by the bones from the bloodstream. (See Suggested Further Reading.)

VOLLEYBALL

This is a good endurance activity for the back, but can cause problems, especially in tall people, who may find that constant *bending* and *arching* is a *strain* on the back.

WALKING

'Walk and be happy, walk and be healthy.'
Charles Dickens, 1812–1870

This is one of the most valuable activities for the back – and it's free! Walking need never involve maximum continuous effort. Start gently and gradually, walking every day, even if it is only for a few minutes.

- Don't stand when you can walk. It is more tiring to stand for a long period than to take a brisk walk.
- When you walk, walk erect, with your bottom tight, stomach pulled in and shoulders back but relaxed, the arms swinging by your sides for *balance*.
- Check your *posture* in a *mirror* before starting your walk.
- Walk with *energy* but in a relaxed fashion, using a 'floating' rhythm. Start easily and work up to a brisk pace which will increase your *breathing* capacity.
- Wear thick soft-soled *shoes*, with a slight heel if necessary to help your balance, and have the knees slightly bent, putting your heel down first, without *jarring* or thumping, each time you take a step.
- Learn to walk lightly, making as little noise as possible.
- If you need gait training, or if you find walking difficult due to bad habits or a disability, then attend a *back school*.
- Walk tall.

Walking can be done virtually at any time, unless the weather is terrible, so put on a good pair of shoes and start walking now.

WARMING UP

This describes *exercises* which warm up the *muscles* and increase the blood flow slowly and gradually, before more vigorous exercise. Long periods need not be spent warming up – a minute or two is sufficient for back exercises. Dancers and *sports* players may take longer in order to prepare the body generally for the greater degree of coordination that is needed. Find your own individual way of warming up before proceeding to more brisk exercise.

WARNINGS

Listen to your body. It will tell you when something is going wrong. If so, heed the warning and stop if you want to avoid *backache*.

WATERBEDS

Many people with bad backs find value in waterbeds since they support every contour of the body in whichever position you lie. The water is displaced by the weight of the body, which means your shoulders, hips and back sink into the mattress. This allows *relaxation* of the back muscles and removes pressure from the back. The addition of heat speeds up the relaxation process and increases the *circulation*.

- They are supportive rather than hard. (See *beds*.)
- They support every contour of the back, hips and shoulders, in whichever *position* you lie.
- They are firm. Modern waterbeds are heavily stabilised so that they feel like a conventional bed.
- A range of mattresses gives you a wide choice, catering for the degree of motion you find most comfortable.

For further details contact the British Waterbed Association. (See Where To Get Help section at the end of the book.)

WATER SKIING

There is a high incidence of injury to the backs of water ski jumpers because the forces involved put an enormous amount of **stress** and **strain** on the back when taking off and landing from a jump. Young water skiers are particularly at risk, so care should be taken with jump heights and boat speeds in order to prevent problems. (See **jarring, vibration**.) People should not be deterred from taking part in this very enjoyable **sport**, but it is more suitable for the mature adult rather than the growing adolescent, unless care is taken and only limited jumping occurs.

WATER THERAPY

See **hydrotherapy**, **swimming**, **thalasso therapy**.

WEAR AND TEAR

See **arthritis**, **degeneration**, **osteoarthrosis**.

WEDGE

The **Putnam** wedge is placed on a horizontal seat and allows you to lean forwards at a table, desk or work surface without putting unwanted **strain** on the back and neck. It allows the back to adjust naturally so that you can maintain a correct upright **posture**. It can thus change any **chair** into a functional therapeutic seat. Furthermore the Putnam wedge has a soft recessed centre which relieves pressure on sensitive areas.

If you need to alter your office chair a wedge is the most inexpensive way of providing an ergonomically sound and medically approved seat for the back, although it is no substitute for a good chair. (See **ergonomics**.)

WEIGHT

'Be fit, not fat.'

If you are overweight you are probably unfit. It is very difficult to weight-watch alone, so join a group. If you have regular activity and **exercise**, with a well-balanced **diet** and the right amount of calories for you, you will be fit.

WEIGHT LIFTING

There are several lifts with graded weights which will increase the strength of the back. The same principles and rules apply as in any **lifting**, but it is advisable to attend a **gym** to learn correct weight lifting techniques.

WHIPLASH

This injury frequently results from a common kind of **car** accident, the rear-end concertina crash. The sudden jerking, **twisting** or whiplash movement of the head on the **neck** in the collision causes stretching and tearing of some of the tissues in the flexible neck, resulting in **pain** and **spasm** on one side. **Muscle** fibres, **tendons**, **ligaments** and nerves may all be damaged, and you may also have a severe **headache**. The sudden scraping which occurs on roughened **joint** surfaces is also extremely painful and provokes muscle spasm immediately as a protective measure. There may even be **locking** of the joints . Small areas of bleeding may occur in the muscle fibres and these may produce permanent **scar tissue**. The medical term for this acute neck condition is torticollis.

What to do

- Always wear a seat belt in the car, and make sure you have properly adjusted head restraints.
- Report the accident at the police station and inform your insurance company, as it may be necessary to make a claim if the injury persists over a period of weeks.

- Lie down with the head well supported and rest. (See **acute back**.)
- Afterwards, wear a neck **collar** for household chores and work, but take it off at regular intervals to prevent **stiffness**.
- Start gentle mobilising movement to prevent the muscles wasting, using your hands to support your head if necessary. Movement will prevent stiffness and more pain.
- See the doctor if the pain persists and there is a constant headache.

WINDSURFING

Repeated **bending** to lift a heavy wet sail out of the water can cause undue strain on the back. It is therefore important not to get tired or begin in heavy seas with a lot of waves and strong winds. Use plenty of **knee** bends to relieve the **strain** on the lower back. (See **squatting**.)

WOOLREST SLEEPER

See **beds**.

WORK

'Work is a four letter word!'

Manual work

The strength needed for manual work varies with the occupation and your body weight. (See **biomechanics**, **levers**.) A big heavy person may only have to lean on something to get it moving, whereas a lighter person may not be able to budge it. However, training and experience provide the skills needed for manual work so it is important that if you are a farmer, a miner, a construction worker, a nurse, a hairdresser or any other manual worker, you know how to push, pull, carry, lift and stand correctly and for how long you are able to maintain the work rate without strain in order to avoid back problems.

(See **carrying**, **ergonomics**, **lifting**, **pushing and pulling**, **standing**.)

Sedentary work

Office workers, machinists and typists are at just as much risk of back pain as manual workers, but for different reasons, such as:

- Badly designed **chairs**.
- Incorrect or varying heights of work surfaces.
- Badly positioned equipment.

Therefore it is important that the workplace is correct for your back. (See **furniture**, **health and safety**, **office**, **visual display unit**.) If you are unhappy about your workplace, discuss it with your personnel officer and your employer or consult one of the other sources of advice.

Redesign your workplace today.

WORRY

Don't worry too much about your back – life in the 20th century is demanding enough as it is. But do try to change your habits and help your back. (See **anxiety**, **help**.)

WRITING SLOPE

A horizontal surface for reading and writing creates back problems for sedentary workers since it encourages forward **bending** of the back, causing **strain** on the **neck** and **lumbar region**. (See **biomechanics**, **ergonomics**.) The use of a writing slope, similar to those used by mediaeval illustrators, Victorian clerks and schoolchildren, provides the **eyes** and the back with a much better distance/angle relationship.

WRY NECK

See **whiplash**.

X-RAYS

An X-ray has two important properties as an aid to the **diagnosis** of back conditions:

- It passes easily through soft structures such as **muscle**, but is stopped by **bone**.
- It darkens photographic paper, so that an X-ray picture, in fact, is the shadow cast by the bone.

X-rays can show up disease and damage in bones and joints, but they will not show up soft tissue damage, for example to **discs, muscles, ligaments** and nerves – for this sort of damage other tests and investigations will have to be made. (See **CAT scan, electromyography, magnetic resonance imaging, nervous system**.)

Ask your doctor why you are having an X-ray or, alternatively, why you aren't having an X-ray. It is your back and every doctor should be prepared to discuss the basics with you. The progress of modern radiation techniques has enabled several pictures to be taken at any one time and bony formation, changes and deterioration in the height of discs can be seen. However, bulging or pressure on a nerve is invisible, so X-rays are not the entire solution. Always ask your doctor what you must do after an X-ray to find out the results – ask questions and insist on answers.

Conditions which show on X-ray

- **Ankylosing spondylitis**.
- **Rheumatoid arthritis**.
- **Spondyloliesthesis**.
- **Scheuermann's disease**.
- **Osteoporosis**.
- **Joint** displacement.
- Crack **fractures**.
- **Paget's disease**.

YANK

This word describes the violent pulling that occurs with a jerk. The back does not like this movement, so if it should occur during treatment or in an activity you may be doing, there is every likelihood that the back will react and there will be discomfort and maybe *pain*.

Care must be taken to distinguish a true yank, which is uncomfortable, and certain techniques which may use a pull. Always choose a qualified registered practitioner for such manipulative treatment. (See *manipulation*.)

YELL

'Nature knows best, and she says, roar.'
Maria Edgeworth, 1767–1849

A shrill cry of pain when a tender area of the back is undergoing *manipulation*, *mobilisation* or *massage* is good. Besides releasing *tension* it will indicate to the practitioner exactly where the site of the problem is. (See *palpation*.) Be positive when you are explaining your back problems as it will enable the practitioner to get you better more easily and quickly.

YIN AND YANG

These are the complementary properties which are brought into balance in the practice of *acupuncture*. According to the ancient Chinese explanation, they control the energy which is the activating force of all phenomena, and they must be in balance to maintain health in an individual.

YOGA

Yoga may have a value in helping backache or in the maintenance of a healthy back. It is a good activity, in that it involves peace of mind through gentle *stretching* and *meditation*, using a series of postures and techniques to help achieve complete physical and mental *relaxation*.

The postures involve the contraction of certain *muscles* and the relaxation of others. In changing from one position to another, previously contracted muscles are relaxed and previously relaxed muscles are contracted, thereby creating muscle strength and endurance, as well as improving muscle relaxation. This all helps avoid back pain.

However, you do need a really good teacher and you must be prepared to learn slowly and carefully, starting with the basic movements. If anything aggravates your back or you lose interest and become ambitious or impatient to learn new postures, you may find yoga is not for you.

YOUTH

People react very differently to back pain. In youth there is usually the attitude that it will go away, but parents should watch carefully to see if back pain occurs during the growing process of their children. (See *observation*.) Parents should be aware of fashion so that back pain does not result. (See *clothing*, *shoes*.) Young people often tolerate pain in order to continue work, to play a sport or to have a good time: conversely, there are also cases of malingering in young people, who wish to avoid exams or some unpleasant task.

ZEAL

'Nothing great was ever achieved without enthusiasm.'

Emerson, 1803–1882

Some people are fanatical about their back and their health. A period of being a zealot might suit everyone with back trouble so that they might, with concentration, understand and resolve their back problems. Then fewer working days would be lost and everyone would be fitter and healthier.

ZERO

No back pain.

ZEST

You cannot have a zest for life with back pain.

ZONE THERAPY

Zone therapy has been practised by the Chinese, Africans and American Indian tribes for thousands of years. The earliest picture is of Egyptian slaves giving it to their masters. It is based on the fact that massage using pressure application on certain parts of the body can relieve discomfort from conditions far removed from where the pressure is applied. (See ***acupressure***, ***reflexology***, ***shiatsu***.)

ZOO

A garden of animals, some of which, like Homo Sapiens, no longer walk on four legs. In order to live in harmony with one another and our environment we should remember that we evolved from moving around on four legs onto two, so from time to time, it is a good idea to exercise on all fours or in a squatting position which may result in a back free from pain.

EPILOGUE

'Look to your health; and if you have it, praise God, and value it next to a good conscience, for health is the second blessing that we mortals are capable of; a blessing that money cannot buy.'

J. Walton

WHERE TO GET HELP

The organisations listed will be able to provide the names and addresses of registered qualified practitioners in your area. Ask your doctor for advice if you are in doubt or not sure which therapy is best for your condition.

Orthodox medicine

Doctors
The British Medical Association
BMA House
Tavistock Square
London WC1
01-387 4499

General Medical Council
44 Hallam Street
London W1N 6AE
01-580 7642

The Royal College of General
    Practitioners
14 Princes Gate
London SW7 1PU
01-581 3232

The Royal College of Physicians
11 St Andrew's Place
London NW1
01-935 1174

Midwives
Royal College of Midwives
15 Mansfield Street
London W1M 0BE
01-580 6523

Nursing
Royal College of Nursing
20 Cavendish Square
London W1
01-409 3333

140

United Kingdom Central Council
    for Nursing Midwifery and Health
    Visiting
23 Portland Place
London W1N 3AF
01-637 7181

Orthopaedics
British Orthopaedic Association
Royal College of Surgeons
35 Lincoln's Inn Fields
London WC2
01-405 6507

Institute of Orthopaedics
234 Great Portland Street
London W1N 5HG
01-387 5070

Institute of Orthopaedic Medicine
81 Belsize Lane
London NW3 5AU

Physiotherapists
The Association of Chartered
    Physiotherapists in Obstetrics
    and Gynaecology
14 Bedford Row
London WC1
01-242 1941

The Chartered Society of
    Physiotherapy
14 Bedford Row
London WC1
01-242 1941

The Manipulation Association of
    Chartered Physiotherapists
14 Bedford Row
London WC1
01-242 1941

The Organisation of Chartered
    Physiotherapists in Private
    Practice
11 The Larches
Benfleet
Essex SS7 4NR
0702 715549

Complementary medicine

Centres of complementary medicine
The British Holistic Medical
    Association
179 Gloucester Place
London NW1 6DX
01-262 5229

The Centre for the Study of
    Complementary Medicine
51 Bedford Place
Southampton
Hants SO1 2DG
0703 334752

The Council for Complementary
    and Alternative Medicine
Suite 1
14/19A Cavendish Square
London W1M 9AD
01-409 1440

The Institute of Complementary
    Medicine
21 Portland Place
London W1N 3AF
01-636 9543

Acupuncture
The British Acupuncture
    Association
34 Alderney Street
London SW1V 4EU
01-334 1012

The British Medical Acupuncture
    Association
15 Devonshire Place
London W1N 1PB

Register of Traditional Chinese
    Medicine
7A Thorndean Street
London SW18 4HE
01-947 1879

Traditional Acupuncture Society
115 Loxley Road
Stratford upon Avon
Worcs CV37 7DS

Alexander Technique
Alexander Research Trust
18 Lansdowne Road
London W11 3LL

Society of Teachers of Alexander
    Technique
10 London House
226 Fulham Road
London SW10 9EL
01-351 0828

Chiropractic
Anglo-European College of
    Chiropractic
13–15 Parkwood Road
Bournemouth
Dorset

The British Chiropractic
    Association
Premier House
10 Greycoat Place
London SW1P 1SB
01-222 8866

European Chiropractors' Union
19 Strawberry Hill Road
Twickenham
Middlesex TW1 4QB

The Institute of Pure Chiropractic
PO Box 127
Oxford OX1 1HH

Faith healers
National Federation of Spiritual
    Healers
Old Manor Farm Studio
Church Street
Sunbury-on-Thames
Middlesex TW16 6R6
0932 78316415

Feldenkrais
The Open Centre
188 Old Street
London EC1
01-278 6783 ext. 3

Herbalism
The National Institute of Medicinal
    Herbalists
148 Forest Road
Tunbridge Wells
Kent

Homeopathy
The British Homeopathic
    Association
27A Devonshire Street
London W1N 1RJ
01-935 2163

The Homeopathic Development
    Foundation
19A Cavendish Square
London W1M 9AD
01-629 3205

Royal London Homeopathic
    Hospital
Great Ormond Street
London WC1
01-837 3091

Society of Homeopaths
47 Canada Grove
Bognor Regis
West Sussex PO21 1DW
0243 860678

The Homeopathic Hospital
Cotham
Bristol 6
0272 731231

The Homeopathic Hospital
600 Great Western Road
Glasgow G12
041-339 0382

Hypnotherapy
London Institute for Clinical
    Hypnotherapy
5 Maddox Street
London W1
01-499 2813

The Register of Psychotherapists
1 Wythburn Place
London W1
01-724 9083
Practitioners trained in
    psychotherapy and
    hypnotherapy.

Manipulation
The British Association of
    Manipulative Medicine
22 Wimpole Street
London W1M 7AD
01-637 0491

The Manipulation Association of
    Chartered Physiotherapists
14 Bedford Row
London WC1
01-242 1941

Massage
The Churchill Centre
22 Montagu Street
Marble Arch
London W1H 1TB
01-402 9475

Clare Maxwell-Hudson
87 Dartmouth Road
London NW2
01-450 6494

East-West Centre
188 Old Street
London EC1
01-251 4076

Naturopathy
The British Naturopathic
    Association
6 Netherhall Gardens
London NW3
01-435 7830

Osteopathy
British College of Naturopathy and
    Osteopathy
6 Netherall Gardens
London NW3
01-435 7830

The British Osteopathic
  Association
8–10 Boston Place
London NW1
01-262 5250

The British Society of Osteopathy
1 Suffolk Street
London SW1Y 4HE
01-930 9254

General Council and Register of
  Osteopaths
21 Suffolk Street
London SW1Y 4HG
01-839 2060/01-930 3889

The Guild of Osteopaths
146–148 Old Oak Road
East Acton
London W3
01-743 5140

Relaxation therapy
Relaxation classes are frequently
run by local authorities. Check with
your local adult education centre.

Yoga
British Wheel of Yoga
1 Hamilton Place
Sleaford
Lincs
0529 306851

East-West Centre
188 Old Street
London EC1
01-251 4076

School of Meditation
158 Holland Park Avenue
London W11
01-603 6116

Scottish Yoga Association
4 Afton Place
Edinburgh EH5 3RB

Yoga Centre of Ireland
Gordon Duffield
10 Clanbrassil Road
Holywood
Northern Ireland BT18 0AR
02317 2782

Yoga for Health Foundation
Ickwell Bury
Biggleswade
Beds SG18 9EF
076 727 271

Yoga classes are frequently run by
local authorities. Check with your
local adult education centre.

Other useful addresses

Age
Age Concern England
Bernard Sunley House
60 Pitcairn Road
Mitcham
Surrey CR4 3LL

Age Concern
Northern Ireland
128 Great Victoria Street
Belfast 2

Age Concern Scotland
33 Castle Street
Edinburgh

Age Concern Wales
1 Park Grove
Cardiff
South Glamorgan

Association of Carers
Medway Homes
Balfour Road
Rochester
Kent ME4 6QU

BASE (British Association for
  Service to the Elderly)
3 Keele Farm House
Keele
Newcastle-under-Lyme
Staffs ST5 5AR

Friends of the Elderly and
  Gentlefolk
42 Ebury Street
London SW1W 0LZ
01-730 8263

Help the Aged
PO Box 460
16–18 St. James's Walk
London EC1
and
1 Seckforde Street
London EC1
01-253 0253

Pensioners Link
17 Balfe Street
London N1 9EB

Pre-Retirement Association
19 Undine Street
London SW17

Pre-Retirement Association
  Resources Unit
Department of Educational Studies
University of Surrey
Guildford GU2 5XH

**Back care products and
furniture**
The Back Shop
24 New Cavendish Street
London W1M 7LH
01-935 9120/9148
Mail order service available.

Beds
The National Bedding Federation
  Ltd
25 Brompton Road
London SW3 2E2

Partners
Tunbridge Wells
Kent TW1 2YZ
0892 43236

See also **Back care products**.

Chairs
See **Back care products**.

Childbirth

The Active Birth Movement
01-221 3833
Exercise classes given by their
members.

The Association of Chartered
  Physiotherapists in Obstetrics
  and Gynaecology
14 Bedford Row
London WC1
01-0242 1941

The National Childbirth Trust
9 Queensborough Terrace
London W2 3T8
01-221 3833

The Royal College of Midwives
15 Mansfield Street
London W1M 0BE
01-580 6523

The Royal College of Obstetricians
  and Gynaecologists
27 Sussex Place
Regents Park
London SW1
01-262 5425

United Kingdom Central Council
  for Nursing, Midwifery and
  Health Visiting
23 Portland Place
London W1N 3AF
01-637 7181

Disability

Banstead Place Mobility Centre
Park Road
Banstead
Surrey
07373 51674

Bristol Aids Centre
172–174 Kellaway Avenue
Horfield
Bristol B56 7YQ

British Amputee Sports Association
2 Bell Road
Cosham
Portsmouth POX 3NX

British Ski Club for the Disabled
Corton House
Corton
Warminster
Wiltshire BA12 0SZ
0985 50321

Central Council for the Disabled
25 Mortimer Street
London W1
01-637 5400

DIAL
National Association of
  Disablement Information and
  Advice Services
117 High Street
Clay Cross
Chesterfield
0246 864498

Disabled Drivers' Association
Ashwellthorpe
Norwich NR16 1RX
050841 449

Disabled Living Foundation
380–384 Harrow Road
London W9 2HU
01-289 6111

John Groom Association for the
  Disabled
Holidays for the Disabled
10 Gloucester Drive
Finsbury Park
London N4 2LP
01-802 7272

Mary Marlborough Lodge for the
  Disabled
Nuffield Orthopaedic Centre
Headington
Oxford OX3 7LD
0865 64811

Riding for the Disabled Association
Avenue R
National Agricultural Centre
Kenilworth
Warwickshire
0203 56107

Royal Association for Disability
  and Rehabilitation (RADAR)
25 Mortimer Street
London W1N 8AB
01-637 5400

Scottish Information for the
  Disabled
Claremont House
18–19 Claremont Crescent
Edinburgh EH7 4QD
031 556 3882

Scottish Sports Association for the
  Disabled
14 Gordon Court
Dalcaverhouse
Dundee DD4 9DL

Sexual Problems for the Disabled
49 Victoria Street
London SW1

Driving

Disabled Drivers' Association
Ashwellthorpe
Norwich NR16 1RX
050841 449

For advice on choosing a car seat
see **Back care products.**

Ergonomics

The Ergonomics Research Unit
The Robens Institute
University of Surrey
Guildford
Surrey GU2 5XH

The Ergonomics Society
University of Technology
Loughborough
Leicestershire LE11 3TU

Exercise

The Aerobic and Fitness Teachers'
  Association
c/o Andre Dean
29 Hursley Road
Chandlers Ford
Hants
04215 3084

The Association of Chartered
Physiotherapists in Exercise,
Recreational and Preventative
Therapy
14 Bedford Row
London WC1
01-242 1941

Keep Fit Association
16 Upper Woburn Place
London WC1 0QG
01-387 4349

The Physical Education
Association
162 Kings Cross Road
London WC1
01-278 9311

Women's League of Health and
Beauty
18 Charing Cross Road
London WC2
01-240 8456

Gym equipment
Bolton Stirland International
Boland House
Nottingham South Industrial Estate
Wilford
Nottingham
0602 822844

Health hydros
Champneys at Tring Ltd
Tring
Herts
04427 3351

Champneys at Stobo
Stobo Castle
Peebleshire
Scotland
0721 6249

Enton Hall
Enton
Godalming
Surrey
042 879 2233

Forest Mere
Liphook
Hampshire
0428 722051

Grayshott Hall
Headley Road
Grayshott
Hindhead
Surrey
042 873 4331

Henlow Grange
Henlow
Bedfordshire
0462 811111

Inglewood Health Hydro Ltd
Kintbury
Newbury
Berks
0488 2022

Ragdale Hall
Ragdale
Melton Mowbray
Leics
066 475 831/411

Shrubland Hall
Coddenham
Ipswich
Suffolk
0473 830404

Tyringham
Newport Pagnell
Bucks
0908 610430

National associations and charities
Arthritis Care
6 Grosvenor Crescent
London SW1X 7ER
01-235 0902

Arthritis and Rheumatism Council
for Research
41 Eagle Street
London WC1R 4AR
01-405 8572

Association for Spina Bifida and
Hydrocephalus
Tavistock House North
Tavistock Square
London WC1H 9HJ
01-388 1382

The National Back Pain
Association
Grundy House
31–33 Park Road
Teddington
Middlesex TW11 0AB
01-977 5474/5
See page 148 for more details of
this association.

National Ankylosing Spondylitis
Society
6 Grosvenor Crescent
London SW1X 7ER
01-235 0902

National Osteoporosis Society
PO Box 10
Barton Meade House
Radstock
Bath BA3 3YB

The British Red Cross
3 Grosvenor Crescent
London SW1X
01-235 3241

The Scoliosis Association (UK)
380–384 Harrow Road
London W9 2HU
01-289 5652

Spinal Injuries Association
76 St James Lane
London N10 3DF
01-444 2121

Pain clinics
Abingdon General Hospital
Abingdon
Berkshire

Royal National Orthopaedic
   Hospital
234 Great Portland Street
London W1N
01-387 5070

Stanmore Orthopaedic Hospital
Brockley Hill
Stanmore
Middlesex

Many other general hospitals now
have pain clinics. Your GP will be
able to advise.

Weight problems

Weight Watchers UK Ltd
11 Fairacres
Bedworth Road
Windsor
Berks
0753 567751

Sport

Sports Council
16 Upper Woburn Place
London WC1H 0QP

Association of Chartered
   Physiotherapists in Sports
   Medicine
14 Bedford Row
London WC1
01-242 1941

Athletics

Amateur Athletics Association
Francis House
Francis Street
London SW1P 1DL
01-828 9326

Badminton

Badminton Association of England
Bracknell Road
Loughton Lodge
Milton Keynes
Bucks
0908 568822

Bowling

English Bowling Association
2a Uddesleigh Road
Dorset BH3 7JR
0202 22233

Cycling

British Cycling Federation
Upper Woburn Place
London WC1 0GE
01-387 9320

Fencing

Amateur Fencing Association
The de Beaumont Centre
Denham Road
West Kensington
London W14 9SP
01-385 7442

Golf

English Golf Union
12a Denmark Street
Wokingham
Berks RG11 2BE
0734 781952

Gymnastics

British Amateur Gymnastics
   Association
5 High Street
Slough
Berks SL1 1DH
0753 32763

Judo

British Judo Association
16 Upper Woburn Place
London WC1H 0QP
01-387 9340

Martial arts

The Martial Arts Commission
Broadway House
15–16 Deptford Broadway
London SE8 4PE
01-691 3433

Parachuting

British Parachute Association
Kimberley House
47 Vaughan Way
Leicester LE1 4SE
0533 59635

Rambling

The Ramblers' Association
1–5 Wandsworth Road
London SW8 1LJ
01-582 6878

Sailing

Royal Yachting Association
Victoria Way
Woking
Surrey GU21 1EQ
04862 5022

Skiing

British Ski Federation
118 Eaton Square
London SW1W 9AF
01-235 8227

Squash rackets

Squash Rackets Association
Francis House
Francis Street
London SW1P 1DE
01-828 3064

Swimming

Amateur Swimming Association
Harold Fern House
Derby Square
Loughborough
Leics LE11 0AL
0509 230431

Table tennis

English Table Tennis Association
21 Claremont
Hastings
East Sussex TN34 1HA
0424 433121

Tennis

Lawn Tennis Association
The Queen's Club
Palliser Road
London W14 9EQ
01-381 4746

Trampolining

British Trampoline Federation Ltd
152a College Road
Harrow
Middlesex

Volleyball
English Volleyball Association
128 Melton Road
West Bridgford
Nottingham NG2 6EP
0602 816324

Water skiing
British Water Ski Federation
16 Upper Woburn Place
London WC1H 0QL
01-387 9371

Weight lifting
British Amateur Weight Lifting
    Association
3 Iffley Turn
Oxford
0865 778319

AUSTRALIA
Australian Chiropractors'
    Association
8 First Street
Murray Bridge
SA 5253
and
1 Martin Place
Linden
New South Wales 2778

Australian College of Rehabilitation
    Medicine
PO Box 341
Ryde
NSW 2112
(02) 807 6771

Australian Council of Allied Health
    Professions
Hospitals Division Health
    Commission of Victoria
555 Collins St
Melbourne
Victoria 3000

Australian Medical Association
77–79 Arundel Street
Glebe
NSW 2037
(02) 660 6466

Australian Orthopaedic Association
229–231 Macquarie Street
Sydney
NSW 2000
(092) 223 3018

Australian Physiotherapy
    Association
25–27 Kerr Street
Fitzroy
Victoria 3065
(03) 417 5244

Australian Society for Medical
    Research
145 Macquarie Street
Sydney
NSW 2000
(02) 27 4461

Australian Society of Teachers of
    the Alexander Technique
    (AUSTAT)
PO Box 529
Milsons Point
Sydney
New South Wales 2061

College of Nursing
Suite 22
431 St Kilda Road
Melbourne
Victoria 3004
(03) 266 5145

Philip Institute of School of
    Chiropractic
Plenty Road
Bundoora
Victoria 3083

CANADA
Academy of Medicine
Box 8223
1867 Alta Vista Dr.
Ottawa ON K1G 3H7
(613) 733 2604

Acupuncture Foundation of
    Canada
7321 Victoria Park Ave.
#302
Markham ON L3R 2Z8
(416) 474 0383

Association of Allied Health
    Professionals
2443 Yonge Street
Toronto ON M4P 2E7
(416) 484 4633

Association of Independent
    Physicians of Ontario
2045 Lakeshore Blvd W.
Toronto ON M8V 2Z6
(416) 259 7034

Canadian Association of Physical
    Medicine and Rehabilitation
    Medicine
339 Windermere Road
London ON NGA 5AS

Canadian Chiropractic Association
1900 Bayview Avenue
Toronto
Ontario M4G 3E6

Canadian Orthopaedic Association
1117 St Catherine St W.
#223
Montreal QCH3B 1H9
(514) 844 9818

Canadian Osteopathic Association
575 Waterloo Street
London ON N6B 2R2
(519) 439 5521

Canadian Physiotherapy
    Association
44 Eglinton Ave W.
#201
Toronto ON M4R 1A1
(416) 485 1139
Branches and/or districts in all
    provinces.

Canadian Podiatry Association
3414 Dixie Road
401 Mississauga
Ontario L4Y 2B1

Canadian Psychiatric Association
225 Lisgar St
#103
Ottawa ONK2P 0C6
(613) 234 2815

Canadian Society of Teachers of
the Alexander Technique
(CANSTAT)
460 Palmerston Boulevard
Toronto
Ontario P7A 4A2

JAPAN
Japan Chiropractors' Association
5-9-3 Chome Kita-Aoyama
Minato-kue
Tokyo

Japan Medical Association
52-Chome Kanda Surugadai
Chiyoda-kue
Tokyo 101

Japanese Physical Therapy
Association
c/o Nimoto Building
2-4-12 Fujami
Chiyoda-kue
Tokyo

NEW ZEALAND
New Zealand Chiropractors'
Association
PO Box 2858
Wellington

The New Zealand Medical
Association
PO Box 156
Wellington

The New Zealand Society of
Physiotherapists Inc.
National Office
PO Box 5198
Lambton Quay
Wellington
and
3rd Floor
Borthwick House
85 The Terrace
Wellington

UNITED STATES OF AMERICA
American Academy of Family
Physicians
1740 W. Ninety-Second Street
Kansas City MO64114

American Academy of Orthopaedic
Surgeons
2010 Massachusetts Avenue NW
Suite 600
Washington DC 20815
(202) 652 0905

American Academy of Orthotists
and Prosthetists
717 Pendleton Street
Alexandria
Virginia 22314
(703) 836 7118

American Association of Colleges
of Nursing
11 Dupont Circle NW
Suite 430
Washington DC 20036
(202) 332 1917

American Association of Hospital
Consultants
1235 Jefferson Davis Highway
Suite 602
Arlington
Virginia 22202
(703) 979 3180

American Chiropractic Association
1916 Wilson Boulevard
Arlington VA 22201

American Medical Association
535 North Dearborn Street
Chicago
Illinois 60611
(312) 751 6000

American Nurses' Association
2420 Pershing Road
Kansas City MO64108
(816) 474 5720

American Osteopathic Association
122C Street NW
Suite 875
Washington DC 20001
(202) 783 3434

American Physical Therapy
Association
1111 North Fairfax Street
Alexandria
Virginia 22314
(703) 684 2782

American Podiatry Association
20 Chevy Chase Circle NW
Washington DC 20015
(202) 537 4900

American Psychiatric Association
1400K Street NW
Washington DC 20005
(202) 682 6000

International Chiropractors'
Association
1901 L Street
NW Suite 800
Washington DC 20036

NATIONAL BACK PAIN ASSOCIATION

The National Back Pain Association is the only organisation in the UK dedicated solely to caring for back pain sufferers. It was founded in 1968. It has several objectives:

- To encourage research into causes and treatment of back pain.
- To help prevent back pain by educating people in the correct use of their bodies.
- To form branches to help back pain sufferers by providing useful information and advice.
- To raise funds to further these objectives.

The NBPA has over 50 branches spread throughout the UK and these are run largely by sufferers on self-help lines, with professional guidance which the Association feels is a most effective means of support.

Research is the most costly of the Association's activities; in 1988 it was supporting projects to the value of approximately £150,000. The research projects are carried out in university departments and hospitals, and the results help provide valuable guidance to consultants, medical practitioners and those who practise complementary medicine. The National Back Pain Association favours a multi-disciplinary approach and is in contact with the many professions involved.

Funding of the Association's work comes entirely from the generosity and benevolence of companies, trusts, private individuals and its membership scheme. Further information can be obtained from The National Back Pain Association's headquarters at:
31–3 Park Road,
Teddington,
Middlesex TW11 OAB.

SUGGESTED FURTHER READING

Back information

The Back: Relief from Pain by Dr Alan Stoddard, Macdonald Optima, London
Examination of the Back by Dr J.K. Paterson and Dr Loic Burn, MTP Press
The Lumbar Spine – An Orthopaedic Challenge by Professor A.L. Nachemson, Lipincott
The Seated Man – Homo Sedens by Dr A.C. Mandal, Dafnia Publications
Total Back Care by Christopher Hayne, Dent, London
Treat Your Own Back by Robin McKenzie, Spinal Publications
Treat Your Own Neck by Robin McKenzie, Spinal Publications
Vertebral Manipulation by Geoffrey Maitland, Butterworths, London

Back therapy

The Alexander Principle by Wilfrid Barlow, Arrow, London
Alexander Technique by Chris Stevens, Macdonald Optima, London
Chinese Medicine: The Web That Has No Weave by Ted Kaptchuk, Cougdon & Weed
Chiropractic by Susan Moore, Macdonald Optima, London.
Osteopathy by Stephen Sandler, Macdonald Optima, London
Manual Therapy for Chronic Headaches by Edeling, Butterworths, London

Childbirth and pregnancy

At Your Best for Birth Eileen Montgomery, John Wright & Sons
Pregnancy Questions Answered Geoffrey Chamberlain, Churchill Livingstone
Preparation for Parenthood Joan McLaren, John Murray

Dance

Ballet Physique by Celia Sparger, Adam & Black
Teaching Young Dancers by Joan Lawson, Adam & Black

Diet

Nutritional Medicine by Dr Stephen Davies, MTP Press
The Arthritis CookBook by Michael McIlwrath, Gollancz, London

Massage

The Complete Book of Massage by Claire Maxwell Hudson, Dorling Kindersley, London

Sport

Keeping the Rider in the Ride (cycling) by Dr W.R. Spence and Michael Sherman
Sports Injuries – a unique guide to self diagnosis and rehabilitation by Dr Malcolm Read and Paul Wade, Cambus Litho

Swimming

Simply Swimming by Molly Houghton, Phoenix Publishing
Aquarobics by Glenda Baum, Faber & Faber, London

Work and communication

Doctor-Patient Communication Edited by Dr David Anderson and McClurg, Academic Press Inc with The Scottish Council of Physical Recreation
Work and Health by Dr Andrew Melhuish, Penguin, Harmondsworth
The Stress Factor by Dr H.E. Stanton, Macdonald Optima, London

Videos

Conquering Back Pain by Champneys and Donald Norfolk, Champneys Group
Mind Your Back by J.C.T. Fairbank MD,FRCS, Videology Ltd

Lifting and Handling by Christopher Hayne, Graves Medical

Available from: The Back Shop, 24 New Cavendish Street, London W1M 7LH
Graves Medical, Holly House, 220 New London Road, Chelmsford, Essex CM2 9BJ
Chattanooga Corporation, Goods Road, Belper, Derbyshire DE5 1UU

BOOKSHOPS

UK

Robinson's Bookshop
11 Bond Street
Brighton

John Wright
44 Triangle West
Bristol

Heffers
Trinity Street
Cambridge

Donald Ferrier Limited
5–18 Teviot Place
Edinburgh

James Thin Booksellers
South Bridge
Edinburgh

John Smith and Son
57–61 St Vincent Street
Glasgow

Austicks Medical Bookshop
57 Great George Street
Leeds

University Bookshop
University Road
Leicester

Parry's Books
Brownlow Hill
Liverpool

Dillons University Bookshop
1 Malet Street
London WC1

W. and G. Foyle
113–119 Charing Cross Road
London WC2

Kimpton's Medical Bookshop
205 Great Portland Street
London W1

H.K. Lewis
136 Gower Street
London WC1

Haigh and Hochland
Oxford Road
Manchester

Thornes University Bookshop
63 and 67 Percy Street
Newcastle

B.H. Blackwell Ltd
48 Broad Street
Oxford

W. Hartley Seed
152–160 West Street
Sheffield

Bowes and Bowes
The University
Highfield
Southampton

Australia

Balding's Book Supplies
50 Edencourt Street
Camp Hill
Queensland 4152

CIG Medishield
202 Berkeley Street
Carlton
Victoria 3053

CIG Medishield
103 Rundle Street
Kent Town South
Australia 5067

CIG Medishield
594 Hay Street
Jolimont
Western Australia 6014

Howden Medical
344 Victoria Street
Darlinghurst
NSW 2010

Surgimed Products Pty Ltd
17 Brisbane Street
Hobart
Tasmania 7000

Canada

University of British Columbia
Book Store
2075 Westbrook Mall
Vancouver, BC V6T 1W5

University of Calgary Medical Book
Store
3330 Hospital Drive N.W.
Health Services Centre
Calgary, Alberta T2N 1N4

University of Alberta Book Store
Students Union Building
88th Avenue–114th Street
Edmonton, Alberta G6G 2J7

McMaster University Medical Book
Store
Chedoke-McMaster Hospital
1200 Main Street West
Hamilton, ON L8N 3Z5

University of Toronto Medical Book
Store
214 College Street
Toronto, ON M5P 3A1

McGill University Medical Book
Store
3655 Drummond Street
Montreal, Quebec
H3G 1Y6

New Zealand

Ackroyd's Medical and Nursing
Books Ltd
PO Box 22-212
Christchurch

Peryer Educational Books Ltd
PO Box 6034
Christchurch

University Bookshop
19 High St
Auckland

University Bookshop
PO Box 6060
Dunedin

Bennetts Bookshop Ltd
PO Box 138
Palmerston North